# Be Healthy, Stay Happy

## A health and happiness book

## (Revised Edition)

## By Ashwini Ahuja

**Published by**

**Kindle Direct Publishing, USA**
**Columbia, SC**

All rights reserved


copyright@ Ashwini Ahuja

For my Healthy family of readers

## A health guide for common people...

Everyone desires to be healthy but don't change lifestyle and unhealthy habits. How to build a relationship between lifestyle and health

Life without healthy lifestyle is a hell....life without beauty is an embarrassment... life that is not happy is a nightmare...and moreover, life without a 'hale and hearty' family is a curse....

## The Author Speaks...

Everyone knows the popular adage: 'a sound mind lives in a sound body'. A sound body, at all times looks attractive and charming. It gives us a sense of real happiness and elation. Needless to say, real beauty comes from within when a person looks properly fit and healthy. An able-bodied and healthy person enhances his personality by putting on chic attires and defines his style statement. Thus, I think Health and Happiness are interrelated. Unhealthy and unfit persons can never think of style. Health contributes to the overall wellbeing in terms of mind, body and social behaviour.

Good health keeps us fine-looking and eye-catching. Inner beauty is the outcome of virtues in you and outer beauty is the result of elegance in style. Thus, health, and happiness are the best components which play an important role in attaining success and admiration in life.  A simple method to become a healthy and fine looking personality is to drink plenty of water and to eat green leafy vegetables and fruits. You can improve your health and increase your happiness by doing regular exercise, aerobics or some yoga etc. So, I think this book is for all those who dream to be healthy and wish to live happy and contented life.

This book is revised edition of previously published "Be Healthy, Stay Happy". It is divided into two sections-

Section One:  Be Healthy

Section Two:  Stay Happy

"Be Healthy, Stay Happy" is a health guide for both men and women. By following the tips in this book, you can make your life healthy and happy and blissful. Don't read this 'guide' like a novel in a single or two sittings. Read a small part regularly then follow the points on a regular basis to discover cent percent results. This book also guides the parents how to cope with the health, perceptive and emotional problems of their preteen kids.

## Index                                              Page

## Chapter One

### Knee Injury: Neglect is More Harmful than Treatment

Knee pain is common among the people of all ages. Although, the elderly people are more prone to this disorder yet the youngsters can also be the sufferers of it caused by their slipshod habits and wide of the mark lifestyle. Curing of the knee injury in time is paramount. Its neglect may be more harmful than treatment.

The protection of knee joint is extremely important for an individual but ironically, these joints are often wounded due to several reasons and people don't take it seriously until they don't have the feelings of throbbing ache. At the time of major knee injury, the pain is very excruciating and unbearable. The patient feels the stiffness in the joints and an acute sensation of inflammation.

Physiotherapist Dr. Pooja Sachdeva Mishra says that "the knee is the joint where thigh bone, shinbone and knee cap hook up. As well, the knee includes cartilage, menisci, ligaments and tendons etc. Cartilage lets the bones rub smoothly over one another when leg bends or it is made straight. Ligaments hold the bones of the knee together and give the knee stability. The menisci are the cushions between the femur and tibia. They act as shock absorbers. Tendons are the connective tissues that connect the muscles to the bones in the leg. When all these components work collectively, the knee remains active". She further says that knee protects the bones from shock and let people to move freely. If you don't take knee pain seriously and have proper treatment, you may be disabling to walk, resulting in handicap".

Dr. Anju Setia, physiotherapist from Shimla says that when the components of knee don't work properly, one can experience pain and inflammation. Here are some treatments to alleviate the knee pain.

## Applying Ice on Ached Knee

If it is knee injury or the pain on the ankle is unbearable, don't delay the treatment. Apply ice immediately and continue this process to three to four times a day. It is the first step for healing. Ice acts as an analgesic. It is good to alleviate the pain and reduce swelling. You can keep the packs or cubes of the ice in a plastic bag or wrapped them in a towel before putting it on ached part of the skin. Direct contact of the ice with the skin is too risky so don't forget to get it covered with towel or plastic bag.

Compression is another option by wrapping with a crepe bandage. Lift the knee by placing pillows below ankle joint. In case of severe pain, lifting weight should be avoided. As for the use of medicine, it should be taken in acute cases of pain. In chronic cases, medicines should also be used whenever there is unbearable pain because the use of medicines continuously causes side effects like hyperacidity and stomach pain.

If you do participate in running or hiking the hilly terrain, be careful and prepared. If you think that you are not at ease in such activities, it is better you quit it or wear kneecap in case you are not quitting it. Before walking briskly or trudging in the hilly area, examine your shoes. Your shoes should be of good quality. They must be cushioned from inside without a bit hard material. High heeled shoes are very risky. Avoid wearing them if you have the feeling of pain around the knees. If there is a difference between your both legs, put insoles in shoes to balance your body posture.

## Body Alignment is Necessary

Those children who have flat feet, knock knees and bowleg problem are very prone to knee or ankle injuries. So, the body alignment is the first step to defend from being the sufferer of knee problem. For body alignment, the parents should be observant. If they are slapdash, their children will have to experience the affliction of ankle pain from time to time. In the early years, parents can prevent their children from these defects. Dr. Anju Setia says that sometimes, these defects disappear itself by the age of 7-8 years. The earlier you intervene, the better you get results.

She further says that before the age of 12-13, the parents may help their children in body alignment with the assistance of physiotherapist. After the age of 13, bones unite. At that time, it is much difficult to overcome the problem without costlier treatment. With the advice of specialists, some sorts of exercises and modification in the shoes, the problem of heel, ankle and knee pain sometimes can be overcome but if you have flat feet, knock knees and bowleg problem, the pain will be arising every so often.

If someone experiences pain in the inner part of the knee, he/she is prone to transfer the weight to the outer part of the leg. As a result, bowleg deformity occurs. If you are suffering from knee arthritis, you are more prone to bowleg deformity due to the shift of the weight from inner part of the leg to the outer part of the leg. Due to bowleg deformity, the shoe heel on the outer side is generally worn out. Dr. Anju Setia furthers that if you want to prevent bowlegs, it is better you go for physical activity and treatment in the form of heel wedge.

## Walking, Posture and Footwear

Walking, posture and footwear play an important role to deal with knee pain. If you wish to walk briskly or do running fast, it is better you prefer smooth and soft flat surface. To prevent from knee injuries, avoid running or walking fast on mountainous terrain. As the age increases, the cushion in the knees becomes degenerated resultantly the legs become feeble. Therefore, elderly people are vulnerable to injury when they experience a mild jerk while walking on rough path.

When you are at work, precisely keep your posture correct. Sit straight. Give proper attention to the chair whilst you are to be seated. The chair should not be excessively low or very high as well to force you bend the joint or struggle you get support for feet. Don't let the knees in flexion for long time. Arrange a chair which is perfect for your height where knees are bent at a comfortable angle and help you to sit down and stand easily. Cross legged sitting is very dangerous if you are prone to knee arthritis.

Wearing proper footwear is also very important but it is generally neglected. Orthopedists generally opine that although people are now aware but we have a long way to go. Walking with wrong or depleted shoes totally negate the benefits of walking. The earlier you replace your worn out and old shoes, the better it might be. Always be careful, the shoes should be able to absorb the shock of the body so as not to put the weight on the ankle and knee joints. Walking shoes should be lighter and soft from inside. They should have possessing sufficient cushions. If you are a regular jogger or runner you must change your shoes after a span of six months. Worn out shoes are more harmful than giving benefits.

## Reduce Weight and Soothing Exercise Routinely

If you are obese, reduce your weight first then think of treatment. Gaining weight is terribly harmful for knee. There are several weight-reducing exercises. The change in lifestyle, regular exercise and eating habits may help you to lose your fat. Obese people are more prone to knee injuries than the slim persons. Dr. Anju Setia says that one kg of extra weight increases six times of the weight on the knees. If an obese person with knee problem doesn't control his weight, he increases the misery to their disability. People suffering from knee pain should stay away from aerobic activities rather they should prefer to stationary cycling or swimming. With aerobic activities, the weight is placed on knee that is very risky.  Also, at home, you can do these exercises:

Sit with your back against the wall. Bend one leg; then straighten it up six inches above the ground. Then slowly and slowly, bring it back. Repeat this activity 10-15 times regularly.

If your leg is severely affected, sit on the floor comfortably; put a pillow under your knee. Push the knee down by tightening the muscles of the leg. Hold for 1-2 minutes. Repeat this exercise 10 times. Apart from these exercises, you may do other exercises like step-up and squats etc.

Dr. Amit Sachdeva of Shimla says that in case of severe instability or pain, you can use knee brace. Although knee wraps are available in the market but they are more damaging than good ones as, by using such wraps, the pressure is increased on the knees. Sometimes, these wraps are too tight to help the ankle; moreover by its constant use, swelling appears on the ankle and its surface appears red.

Dr. Amit Sachdeva suggests it is better if you use knee support or brace when you have a feeling of pain or instability because knee brace has a hole in the centre for patella (knee cap). If you have a severe and unbearable pain, then analgesic ointment is good for temporary treatment. It increases the temperature by generating heat in the area making the patient relaxed but it has no healing effects, whatsoever.

## POINTS TO REMEMBER

Too much rest can weaken your muscles worsening the joint pain.

Rest, ice, compression and elevation are good for knee pain due to minor injury. Give your knee some rest, apply ice to lessen pain and swelling. Wear crepe bandage. Keep the knee elevated.

Use handrails while you go upstairs. Use strong ladder or foot stool to get something from high shelf.

Control your weight. If you are overweight, reduce it. Losing weight will lessen the stress on your knees.

Do traditional Chinese way of treatment: Acupuncture and Tai Chi. Sure enough, these ways will help you ease stiffness and improve balance. In acupuncture treatment, needles are inserted at certain points in the body for relief in pain.

Use cushioned insole to reduce stress on your knees.

Avoid jarring exercise viz. jumping, jogging, running and kickboxing.

Six foods are excellent for knee health:   Soya, Fish, Avocado, Flaxseeds, Berries, Ginger

Vitamin C is best for knees. Use maximum vitamin C to keep your knees in shape.

Reduce alcohol intake and give up smoking to reduce the disorders that lead to knee pain.

Maintain good sleeping habits. Go to bed in time and wake up early in the morning.

Sleep in comfortable position, with a pillow between your legs.

Use good quality, firm mattress with a foam cushion on its top to help distribute your weight.

Avoid higher dose of medicine regularly to kill the pain or to have a good sleep.

Proper stretching is necessary. Physical activity without proper stretching can put you at risk for a traumatic knee injury. If you are feeling pain, avoid playing intense sports like basketball and football.

Avoid falling from the height. There are chances of traumatic injuries.

Check your metabolism regularly. If the rate is not positive, do it right after consulting the doctor. Metabolism disorder connects to chronic knee pain.

Gout is the result of metabolic disorder and it often experiences knee pain.

## Chapter Two

### Sedentary Life Style:

### Major Cause of Varicose Veins!

Have you heard about varicose veins? In the past, nobody heard about it. But, these days, this problem has become commonplace. A report says that today, almost twenty percent people of India are suffering from varicose disease. Among them, women are prone to four times more than their counterparts.

Dr. Amit Sachdeva, Senior Resident, Department of Community, Medicine, IGMC; Shimla says that modern fashion, comfortable and sedentary life is the root cause of this disease.

Young female who wear tight jeans and high heeled sandals are more prone to varicose veins. Except for it, ladies prefer to stand while cooking or household chores in kitchen are more victim of this syndrome.

In professional life, the more use of computer and special posture, while performing duties, has increased the incidence of varicose vein.

Today, men and women working at counters in mall shops and department stores, computer professional, salesmen, receptionists, traffic police, security guards are the worst sufferers of varicose veins.

### What is Varicose Vein?

When veins beneath the skin of legs and thigh become widened, enlarged, swollen and twisted, they are called varicose veins. Varicose veins are actually abnormal veins. These veins are knotted tightly, looks as if a group of blue or purple worms or snakes sitting beneath the leg.

The function of the valves is to control the blood flow in the veins. The problem happens when valves become defective and allow the flow of blood in wrong direction. Briefly, in these veins, when the impure blood from the lower part back to the heart gets disordered due to effective valves of the reins, the normal veins turns into varicose veins.

Due to standing for long time or wearing high heeled shoes or tight outfits, the overload of pressure affects the function of the veins. And the problem of varicose veins starts. With its start, swelling and heaviness in the feet are visible and patches of blue colour begin to develop under the skin of leg. Resultantly, the shape of leg and foot become distorted. If the problem persists for long time, the patient is forced to lead a disabled life.

There are two main types of veins in the legs - deep veins and superficial veins. When leg muscles squeeze the deep veins at the time of walk wearing tight dress and high heeled shoes, it is known as deep veins type. In deep veins type, most of the blood carries back up the legs to the heart. These veins are far from the surface of the body while superficial veins are close to the surface of the body.

In brief, superficial veins are not as important as the deep veins but you can not ignore them if the problem persists. It is said that, In USA, one in four adults is affected by varicose veins.

## Varicose Veins: Origin of the Disease

The disease of varicose veins relates to the flow of blood in the veins of legs. When blood doesn't flow properly through the legs' veins, the disease develops. Normally, when you are healthy, blood flows from the superficial veins to the deep veins then from there it flows back up to the heart. One way flaps or valves in these veins make sure that the blood flows in right direction. If one or more valves leaks, blood may route the wrong path from deep veins to superficial veins.

In such a case, leg is under more pressure. Leg muscles contract and the valves inside the veins open making the legs swell and bulge. In such a situation, the disease of varicose veins start. It happens when one is in the upright position. The blood in his/her leg veins then work against the gravity to return to the heart.

## Causes of Varicose Veins

Doctors generally say that the problem of varicose veins is genetic. If your parents have the problem of varicose veins, there are higher chances you are prone to it. In fact, the disease passes from one family or generation to other family or generation. Lack of exercise, overweight of body, old age, obesity; abnormal life style, excess pressure on veins, prolonged standing and sitting with legs dangling down - are several reasons to varicose veins.

As the age increases, the risk of varicose veins enhances. Ageing erodes the valves in veins that help control the flow of the blood. In old age, when body gains weight, the valves fail to flow the blood up to the heart because overweight puts added pressure on the veins. This disease is more common in patients who are tall.

Among ladies, the problem of varicose veins is common. A hormonal change during pregnancy, puberty, menopause or post pregnancy periods is the factor as female hormones have a tendency to relax vein walls.

The ladies who consume birth control pills are more prone to risk of varicose veins. Due to lack of exercise, veins of legs become very weak and develop into varicose at later stage. Due to obesity, a big quantity of fat gets deposited in the legs which harms the veins.

Dr. Anju Sachdeva of Shimla opines that apart from high heeled sandals and jeans, tight belts and panties are also the significant reason to the development of varicose veins. The items which obstruct the normal flow of blood in veins are actually the causes of varicose veins.

She further says that arteries pass on blood from your heart to the rest of your tissues. Veins return blood from the rest of your body to your heart. This way, blood is re-circulated. To push blood to your heart, the veins in your legs must have the power to work against gravity. When the power diminishes, the problem of varicose veins occurs.

**Varicose Veins: Symptoms**

Leg feels heavy and aching especially after an exercise

Veins or ankles look swollen, bulging and gnarled.

A minor injury to the affected area resulting longer bleeding

The colour of the veins is blue, brownish or dark purple.

When suddenly standing up, one experiences leg cramps.

Inflammation of the skin

Hardening of the vein

Skin ulcers close to ankle

Itching on one or more veins

Weakness and discomfort in the knees

Inability to stand properly or fully stretching out the knee. Popping of sounds as the knee bends or straightens out

Swelling and stiffness on the knee

Reddishness and heated sensations

Types of Varicose Veins

There are three main types of varicose veins.

Trunk Varicose Veins

Reticular Varicose Veins

Spider Varicose Veins

Trunk varicose veins are close to the surface of the skin. They are thick and knotted. They look unpleasant and disgusting. Reticular varicose veins are red in colour. They are clustered close together. Spider varicose veins are known as thread veins. They look like a group of small spiders. They are a small group of red or blue veins every so often appear on face or legs.  Spider veins are harmless. They don't swell beneath the surface of the skin.

## Varicose Veins: Self Care

If the disease of varicose veins is in its initial stage, you can ease its pain through self care methods such as moderate exercise and wearing compression stockings. Such methods, for the time being, are good ones but these can't cure your disease completely without the application of medication. To prevent your health from getting worse, you must contact the specialist doctor. Self care measures are good at initial stage.

Ulcers and blood clots close to varicose veins particularly near the ankles are indications that disease requires immediate attention. Ulcers are caused by fluids collected inside the tissues for the long time. It is caused by increased pressure of the blood within the affected veins. Before the origin of an ulcer, usually; a discoloured spot on the skin appears.

In such a situation, immediately contact the doctor. If you have a sudden swelling on leg regularly, chances of the blood clot are there. In such situation also, you may also be long-suffering of the disease.

## Varicose Veins: Precaution and Prevention

Precaution and prevention are always a better option to stay away from any disease. There is no way to absolutely prevent varicose veins but if you improve your blood circulation and improve your muscle tone, you can reduce the risk of developing varicose veins. If you have already a victim of the disease, then there is no other option except the application of medication but if you are fine, these methods at home can help you prevent the disease.

### Go for exercise regularly.

Don't miss the morning walk

Keep checking your weight.

Prefer to eat high fiber diet.

Keep changing your posture while working at office.

Keep elevating your legs. Don't cross them while sitting.

Avoid excess salt in diet.

Always be active, energetic and happy

Avoid wearing high heels for long time

Before getting out of the bed in the morning, put on socks.

Keep wearing the socks all day. It would prevent blood from amassing in your legs.

Always sleep on left side. It can help prevent varicose veins.

## Specialists' Views

Recently, in a two day symposium at Chandigarh on the subject 'Innovative Treatment of Varicose Veins' Professor A. K Attri and Dr. Ravul Jindal, Vascular Surgeon, Fortis opines that lack of proper knowledge among medicos regarding varicose veins often leads to aggravation of problem.

Due to lack of knowledge, the appropriate treatment is delayed and the patients have to undergone excruciating pain. Dr. Jindal further says that varicose veins need to be treated as early as it is diagnosed. At the early stage, disease can be controlled through medicines but if it is delayed, surgery is required to eliminate varicose ulcer.

If truth be told, people of our country are quite unaware of this disease. Patients of varicose veins generally visit general surgeon or physician. Sometimes, this disease is misconstrued bone problem, arthritis or skin disease.

Dr. Jindal suggests that in case a bit of suspicion arises, don't hesitate to consult cardiovascular surgeon instead of general surgeon.

## Varicose Veins: Numerous Misconceptions

One of the biggest misconceptions regarding varicose veins is that it is a disease of an old age.  Remember, though you are quite young but your habits are not fine, to a certain extent, your lifestyle is unhealthy, you maybe the victim of varicose veins. Varicose veins can develop even at the age of 10 years or less. It is linked with heredity, not age.

If both parents have the history of varicose veins, it is guaranteed that at some point in your life, you will be the victim of this disease. Therefore, get rid of the biggest misconception that it is a disease of an old age.

**Second misconception:** varicose vein is the problem of women only; men are not at risk. No, it is a myth. Several reports say that more than fifty percent men are affected by varicose veins. They felt pain and itchiness similarly as their ladies counterparts. They too have the excruciating experience of burning, throbbing, muscle cramping and swelling in any part of their legs.  Generally, varicose veins are found in thighs and calves but sometimes, they can also be found on the face.

**Third misconception:** varicose vein is just cosmetic. There is no need of treatment for it. It may be the quack's bad advice. Don't believe such counseling. Sometimes, patients feel no pain in spite of the clear symptoms of varicose veins. Despite that, the advice of the experts is essentially required. Carelessness may lead to increase the disease resulting in more serious damage to the body such as leg ulcers and heart failure.

**Fourth misconception:** it is said that the treatment of varicose veins is too expensive. As it is considered as a cosmetic treatment so, most of the health insurance companies don't cover it in their plans. It is erroneous information. It is clarified, when the treatment of varicose veins is done for medical reasons i.e. treatment of symptomatic varicose veins - swelling, ulceration, bleeding veins, tired legs etc., it is covered by numerous insurance companies but the removal of spider veins which is usually done for cosmetic reasons is not covered.

## Non Surgical Treatment of Varicose Veins

Compression Stockings

Ablation Therapy

Sclero Therapy

The first and foremost treatment for varicose veins is compression stockings. In the early period of the disease, knee-high compression stocking is the best treatment. It helps relieve in pain and swelling. Compression stockings compress the veins and check blood from travelling down pooling in the legs. Even the requirement of the health insurance companies is that the claimant should wear compression stockings for at least three months before going for surgery type major treatment.

When compression stockings don't give sufficient relief to patients, some form of ablation therapy such as laser, mechanical injection and radio frequency is applied to relax the affected veins. Before the ablation therapy, leg is cleansed and sterile drapes are placed.

After that, the doctor gives the injections to numb the area so as he could insert a thin tube into the vein after a small cut. The tube is pressed forward into the entire vein and all the surrounding skin is anesthetized but the patient is awake during the all process of the therapy.

This is called ablation catheter or therapy. In this therapy varicose veins are heated either by radio waves or a laser. Ablation procedures are generally invasive alternatives to traditional surgery for varicose veins. It is painless procedure and takes less than half an hour. Usually, doctors offer this treatment to the patients first. Subsequently, the leg is wrapped with a compression bandage.

In sclerotherapy, a foam like chemical namely sclerosant is injected into veins through a small needle. When the affected veins are not pretty straight, surgeons prefer sclerotherapy. In this therapy, the patients need two to three sessions of treatment. After the treatment varicose veins disappear. It is less invasive than surgery. Even the treatment of small spider veins is also done in the same way by using a tiny tube or needle into the affected veins.

## Chapter Three

### How to Boost Your Immunity?

When the season is changed after a spell of rain, our immune system gets worsened. That time, we are susceptible to several ailments. Bio-chemistry of our body changes, sweat oozes; we lose salt and water of the body which affects our immunity system. In changed weather, viruses also become more active resulting to ailing the body.

Dr. Ravindra Lavania says that in such weather, cold and cough are common diseases. If you are careless, you can invite malaria, diarrhea, sore throat, upset stomach, asthma, dengue, typhoid, joint pain etc. also These all are allergy related conditions which can be overcome by boosting body's defence mechanism or immunity to fight germs and bacteria.

### What is Our Immune System?

Dr. Suneer Thakkar says that a collection of organs, cells and antibodies whose purpose is to defend our body against several diseases is immune system.

It is our defence mechanism against prevalent infections. There are several factors that weaken our immune system which prevent our body from fighting the viruses. Weakened immune system is an enemy to health; so always try to boost your immunity to fight against diseases.

## In the Favor of Vitamin C

Dr. Suneer Thakkar opines that if you are first exposed to illness, you must start to take vitamin C to make stronger your immune system and continue taking it until the risk is over. Dr. Ravindra Lavania says that vitamin C work as an antioxidant which allows the body to flush out waste and bacteria. Antioxidants normally help the body to function better. It should be taken in its purest form.

## How to Boost Body Defence Mechanism

Dr. Amit Sachdeva suggests some ways to boost the body defence mechanism.

Compensate body's salt and water which is lost due to sweating by having plenty of fluids viz. soup and simple water. They will help you flush out the body's waste and germs.

Take sufficient juice but don't resort to roadside stalls or kiosks for it.

Vitamin C is the best source to boost the immunity so take *nibbu paani* without sugar two times a day minimum.

You can also take orange and lemonade.

In this weather, avoid chaat, sliced fruits, gol gappas etc. from *rehris* or eating outside because these uncooked items attract microbes.

Eat fresh and healthy salad and fruits at home.

Don't step out from an AC car into hot sun instantly.

If you feel joint pains or osteoarthritis, don't walk in the sun.

It is better if you exercise regularly to avoid stiffness in the joints.

Eat each meal on time. Never skip them. It is the only proper all time-meal which helps you maintain your immunity.

To control the cold and cough at the earliest stage, you must consult your doctor and take prescribed antibiotics.

Doctor can also prescribe you some supplements to boost your immune system.

Moreover, adopt a healthy lifestyle. Shun smoking, drinking and excessive caffeine as well.

Don't work for long hours. If necessary, take rest in the intervening time.

If you haven't been immunized. Do the vaccination to both children and adults at this time to shield your health.

Yogurt also helps to build immunity. Take it if doctor advises.

Green Tea has dual immunity building purpose. It works as an antioxidant as well as strengthen our body system. Moreover, green tea has more cell rebuilding properties than both white and red tea.

To keep your body fit and fine, do regular exercise. It will increase your blood circulation and also burn off your fats and sweat out toxins etc. Obese people often reduce immunity.

Have a plenty of sleep. Laugh with cracks. Dr. Suneer Thakkar says that laughter helps the body release endorphins which help the body healthy and feel us better.

Last but not least, think positively and distress yourself for always.

## Chapter Four

### How to Flatten Your Tummy?

Stomach is the most challenging area in our body. We all want our stomach gets flattened overnight. For this, we, despite having our busy schedule, crazily perform hundreds of crunches, sit ups; leg lifts etc. to burn off extra fat and calories but stomach seems unyielding and getting in shape.

Moreover, we stick on consuming sugar free and low carb diets also which are easily available in market but we see no better results. Where is the slipup?

Delhi based dietician Dr. Rekha Sehgal says that most of us are ignorant both about right food schedule and accurate exercises. We all exactly don't know what we need to lose our tummy fat.

Without the guidance of both the dietician and the health coach, we will find no good results. Remember, we can't lose fat from a specific body part by doing fixed exercises. People need to focus on exercises which burn the most body fat especially cardio workouts and full body weight training.

Moreover, most market- available foods which labeled as sugar free or low carb are not good for health. They actually contain artificial sweeteners, sugar alcohols and other additives but people trust on them. Actually, these diets too don't yield better results.

Before taking such foods, consultation with the dietician is mandatory; Dr. Rekha advises, otherwise some such types may create hormonal mess inside the body resulting in more fats in spite of flattening.

She further says if the purpose of anyone is only to thin the waistline and fine flat tummy, they should adopt the combination of strength training focusing on tummy, cardiovascular exercise and stable blood sugar keeping away from additional fat and sugar.

If one wants to shed the stubborn flab unbelievably in short period and make the waistline sexy and slim-dim, remember some dietary tricks and workout techniques.

Boost your metabolism to burn your fat. For this, jogging or running at least 30-40 minutes is the best option.

Do running or jogging at least four days a week to get result in short period.

Drink skimmed milk necessarily.  Avoid white bread, potatoes & white rice for minimum three days a week.

Eat fresh fruits and green vegetables regularly.

Focus on brown rice and wheat bread.

Avoid diary products viz. butter, ghee, cheese etc. and red meat to get rid of bloating and gas.

Protein helps in burning fat. Almond is the best source to get protein. Eat at least five six almond daily at morning time. It is known as the healthiest snack in the present time.

Go to gym three days a week- minimum and concentrate on your middle section apart from cardio.

Never eat anything at bedtime.

Drink plenty of water regularly. It will help you in digestion as well as fill you up so as you could eat less.

Drinking water empty stomach also helps reducing the fat.

Don't focus on traditionally two three times meals. Extend it four five times. It will help kicking up metabolism.

Don't change your routine. Remain consistently with your exercise routine and diet.

If you are irregular at diet, abdominizer machines or rocker-roller-lounger also can't help you a little.

Avoid consuming "fat burner pills" available in the markets and save your precious money.

You can increase your metabolism by cycling, swimming or stair climbing etc.

Repeat every exercise 5-7 times taking two three minutes recovery time of catch breath.

Remember one most important point: never starve yourself, eat sensibly and right things to tone your body. If you eat poorly, no amount of workout will help you.

## Chapter Five

## How to Mitigate the Severe Migraine Attack?

Are you the patient of migraine? Do you understand why you always fail to find out the reasons of your severe headache? Most of us who are the sufferers of migraine just consume one or two heavy painkillers and, anyhow, try to mitigate the migraine pain. Is it the right way to cure the disease? Doctors opine that there are several reasons to headache but nothing is worse than migraine attack. It is one of the most agonizing experiences as one is completely helpless and no doctor can stop the migraine's severe pain immediately.

## WHAT IS MIGRAINE?

Dr. Amit Sachdeva says that it is a painful neurological condition. The most common symptom of migraine is severe episodic headache. With migraine attack, head on its half spins like a wheel and body convulses becoming the life halt. Normal painkillers like ibuprofen and nimesulide don't help to mitigate the pain. Heavy painkillers just numb the pain for sometime. But, it is not the proper and right treatment.

Migraine leads to high blood pressure. Also, it elevates the level of cholesterol in the body. So, it should not be considered a minor ailment. Although, migraine has nothing to do with cardiovascular diseases yet its constant pain can also become the cause of cardiac arrest or high blood pressure.

## WHY MIGRAINE STARTS

Migraine starts when you are worried over a situation which you don't want to face or accept. Such situation can affect on your body and mind. If you don't find its solution immediately, it may become serious health problem at later stage giving birth to painful migraine. Sometimes, we think that we are not in anxiety but even its constant low level also can give birth to migraine.

Dr. Madhu Sharma says that before the onset of the migraine, we have a feeling of light flashes, blurred vision and formation of dazzling zigzag lines before the eyes. Sometimes, constant smoking, obesity and high cholesterol can also become the reason of migraine. Dr. Anju Sachdeva says that there is no single cause of migraines. Depression, worry, sour food, intestinal inflammation, constipation, constant work on computer and TV watching are the main reasons of migraine, she adds. Genetic and hormonal factors play an important role triggering the migraine attack.

## HOW IS MIGRAINE DIAGNOSED?

Dr. Arun Makker, MD says that there is no specific test to diagnose migraine headache. If the patient experiences recurring headache, the doctor can advise him/her to keep the record of pain in a diary and the symptoms leading to headache, then he can ascertain if there is really a migraine headache. The doctor may also ascertain whether such headaches also run in your family. There are several reasons of severe headache. Every severe headache is not migraine.

## HEALTHY LIFESTYLE CAN HELP

Dr. Anju Sachdeva opines that most migraine sufferers try to control the pain by taking strong painkillers. It is not a healthy practice. Its constant use has enormous power to create hazardous side effects on kidney and liver. It is better if you adopt the healthy lifestyle plus over-the-counter medicines simultaneously. Healthy lifestyle is: sound sleep, balanced diets and regular exercise. Healthy lifestyle alleviates tension, stress and anxiety. It helps to boost the immune system. It is most important because we know that it is only stress which triggers the migraine attack.

Dr. Amit Sachdeva also says that people generally throw their problems under carpet thinking that they will disappear routinely but it never happens. The problems later become the cause of hyper tension and anxiety which invite several ailments which weaken our immune system. Migraine is common among such people. It is the only healthy lifestyle and the timely solution of every problem which help us to control the migraine.

## OTHER TREATMENTS

Dr. Ajay Grover, an Ayurvedic practitioner says that acupuncture, massage, hypnosis are the best medications of migraine. Feverfew medicine which is manufactured by deriving the essence from a plant of sunflower family can also prove a boon for the patients of migraine.

Dr. Suneer Thakkar says that every disease and dysfunction in the body is psychosomatic. The roots of every problem in the body directly connect to mind so always keep your mind in peace. The doctors should advise the patients to take safer drugs in consideration of high blood pressure, high cholesterol and variety of cardiovascular diseases.

Dr. Ravindra Lavania says that if you are mentally disturbed or stressed, it will affect your sleep and appetite leading to have an effect on your immune system also. When one's immune system is weak then body becomes an easy target for viruses and bacteria so, the main reason of the multiple diseases in body is our disturbed immune system.

Dr. Lavania cautions that middle age people should always be extra alert. If they are suffering from migraine, they are more at risk of heart attacks or cardiovascular diseases. They should always keep their immune system in check.

## SOME TIPS TO MITIGATE MIGRAINE HEADACHE

First, try to know if you are really the patient of migraine, then the solution of the problem is not hard to find with healthy lifestyle.

Always do regular morning walk or physical exercise.

Yoga and meditation can also diminish tension and stress.

Join gym or run in the ground to channelize your energy in a positive direction.

Always be free of worries and unnecessary thoughts.

Yoga experts advise that if you are patients of migraine attack, practice *sahaj pranayama*. In this yoga asana, you should sit quietly with eyes closed and doing nothing. You relax yourself completely and try to understand your mental problem.

Avoid late sleeping, spicy and stale bakery food.

Lie down and take rest in a darkened and quiet room if pain becomes unbearable.

Have a cold pack on your head to comfort your pain.

Take multi vitamins tablets or any other supplements under doctor's prescription. Doctors say that sometimes magnesium deficiency can also become the reason of migraine. Consult the doctor to find out the reason of headache.

Dr. Amit Sachdeva suggests if you are prone to uncontrolled problem, ask the doctor for EMG training except for the Imitrex the best medication of migraines.

## Chapter Six

### How to Protect Your Kids' Teeth

Parents are generally anxious over the protection of their kids' teeth. Essentially, you must have been one of them. We all know that as the child grows, he starts to eat repeatedly and the parents delight in having seen their kids eating even after short intervals and they don't stop him from frequent munching.

A few parents know that the problem of early childhood dental cavies arises just after the teeth make their appearance in child's mouth. Parents generally think that the baby teeth are temporary and are going to fall out after a period then why they worry about them? Actually, it is not the truth.

Dr. Meenakshi Kataria, a dentist says that these teeth play an important role in child's health and development because they enable the kids to chew the food properly and also help them to pronounce the all new words at the time of learning at school.

Moreover, early decay of kids' teeth can lead to permanent teeth growing in the crooked shape which distorts the attractive smile of the kids and reduce the beauty of their faces.

Thus, if you want your kids' permanent teeth grow in proper shape, you must care for them since the birth of your baby child.

## Before the Appearance of First Tooth

Generally, the first tooth of a new born baby comes at about six month of age. At the time of baby's birth, the oral cavity has only gum pad. Most parents don't care about the gum pad as they think that the baby takes only liquids- breast feeding or the drops of water etc. so there is no chance of decay in the mouth.

Dr. Meenakshi Kataria opines that the parents should start caring for the baby's oral hygiene right after its birth by proper cleaning of the gum pads from time to time by a wet piece of soft cloth.

As soon as any tooth appears in the mouth, parents should wipe it clean carefully. For it, piece of damp cotton can also be used. When the five six teeth erupt, the parents should assist their kids to brush the teeth regularly until they learn to use the brush on his own effectively.

## Don't Share Spoon with the Baby

Most parents share utensils with their children when they look after them. This way, the bacteria which enter in kids' mouth is because of parents' negligent behavior. There are several mothers who clean the spoon of the baby with their tongue or taste everything before giving it to their children.

This way, they are responsible entering the bacteria in child's mouth. So, never clean the spoon with your tongue by licking it. It is a source of transmitting infection to the child. Kissing the child onto the lips also transmits infection.

## Check the Thumb Sucking Habit

Thumb sucking is common practice among tiny kids. By the age of three four year, it is all right but some children don't stop sucking their thumbs after that age and parents don't care about the bad habit of their children.

If your more-than-four-year child sucks thumb discourage him forthrightly. Thumb sucking habit can lead the mouth deformation and tooth alignment.

## Excessive Feed and Sugar Causes Dental Caries

Most children love to eat sugary items. It also causes cavities. Don't allow your kids to eat sugary items more than five times a day. Dr. Anju Setia says that the frequency of intake of sugar stuff matters more than the amount of sugar consumed.

Epidemiologic studies show that the intake of meals (not only sugar) more than five times a day also leads to an increase in the number of cavities.

Dr. Meenakshi Kataria says when the child begins to weep most women thrust their breast feed into the mouth of the child without knowing the actual reason of the weeping. Such practice also leads to childhood dental caries.

Breast feeding should also be given at proper hours not only for the dental health of the baby but for the overall health of the child.

## When Baby is under Two year

1    Never lay your baby on bed with a bottle in his mouth. It can deform the teeth shape. Help him/her while he/she takes feed.

2    Make sure the bottle is clean and dry.

3    Do not dip the pacifier in honey to delight the baby when he/she is weeping. No doubt, children like sweet taste but its excessive use will cause tooth decay. Germs in honey can also make the child sick.

4    Clean the nipples of bottle every time by washing with soap, rinsing carefully with clean water.

## Don't Ever Forget

Inculcate the habit of brushing in your child by brushing your teeth before them twice a day.

Teach them the proper way of brushing.

Don't let your child swallow tooth paste. You dispense the toothpaste themselves and also supervise brushing until the child is seven-eight year old.

Teach your child not to take sugary items or drinks frequently because tooth decay is caused by bacteria in the mouth interacting with sugar.

Use fluoridated toothpaste immediately after the child learns to spit toothpaste out.

## Chapter Seven

### Mud Therapy: Natural Wellness to Human Body

In ancient Vedas, we not only find the mention of mud or earth and its plentiful benefits but various methods of treatment by mud are also defined in these voluminous epics. At present, mud therapy is known as a best one relaxing experience to the ailing body without any side effect. It is best known as an integrated and well acknowledged therapy of naturopathic science rendering a number of health improving benefits, which in the long run imparts natural wellness to human body.

Since the ancient times, mud therapy is being used to cure several chronicle diseases by the Ayurvedic practitioners. It is regarded as one thousand year old traditional Indian natural treatment. It has proved that in the treatment of several diseases, mud therapy is even better than allopathic treatment. No doubt, the earth has numerous healing powers. Thus, mud therapy is a refreshing and invigorating experience for the body. It is best for natural wellness to human body.

Indeed, this ayurvedic therapy is based on the principals of two elements- the earth and the air. Doctors strongly believe that the mud has a plentiful medical property for all kinds of diseases. In old times, our ancestors residing in villages have mud coating on the inner and outer of their houses to keep them cool during summer and warm during winter. That way, they also keep the diseases and germs outside the houses. The best point in mud therapy is: it has no side effect as in allopathic medicines while using them.

Even several allopathic practitioners believe that mud therapy is more effective treatment than allopathic in some incurable diseases such as migraine, asthma, indigestion, arthritis, viral infection, paralysis, spondylitis, mental disorder and sinusitis etc. It also gives better results regarding general health and wellbeing. Ayurvedic practitioners say that soil of northern hills is good for arthritis, paralysis and spondylitis and mud of the desert is known as a boon for viral infection.

It is believed that the concept of mud therapy is originated from South India so, southern part of India is known for its best medicinal properties. It is also believed that southern mud is rich in minerals and several other effective properties.

## Good for General Wellbeing

In the age of hectic lifestyles, mud therapy is undoubtedly a fine, an effective and result-oriented treatment for the general health of human beings. Not only in India, people from western countries are also tending to alternative medicine systems. They are now aware about the side effects of allopathic treatment. They have now woken up to the possibilities of its (alternative medicine systems) efficacy. So, in western countries, naturopathy such as oil massage therapy, magnetic therapy, herbal therapy, music therapy, aromatherapy, acupuncture apart from best result-oriented mud therapy are gaining popularity day by day.

Dr. David Eisenberg a surgeon at "Centre for Alternative Medicine" Harvard says that now Americans are spending billions on alternative medicine to explore all possible avenues. Although Ayurveda is more than five thousand year old but they people always remained unsuccessful in recognising its effectiveness. Now they are aware about its benefits.

At present, not only the common people, even celebrities like Naomi Campbell, Madonna and Demi Moore too began to love India's ancient science for treatment. Gopi Warrier, an Indian and the first founder of "Ayurvedic Charitable Hospital" in Britain has once said that in contrast to western allopathic medicine, the Indian Ayurveda has an excellent record of curing the several kinds of chronic problems. Whether it is the migraine or the enzema, Ayurveda can reach to the root of every problem.

## A Boon for Skin Rejuvenation

Mud is known the best medicine for skin, body and mind rejuvenation. When it is mixed with chandan, it emerges as one of the best beauty secrets. It is believed that it calms down the senses. It removes the wrinkles and retains the moisture of the body intact. It opens the pores of the skin relieving internal pain and congestion.

It increases the beauty of the skin. Mud therapy helps us in clearing the dark spots and patches on our face. It improves our complexion. It is also helpful for those who are suffering from heat or burn. It also helps the patients suffering from diseases like leucoderma, rheumatic pain and leprosy. Any pain due to injuries is also calmed down by mud application.

It is also a good method for the treatment of skin diseases of every kind. Doctors say that wet clay absorbs toxins in the skin. So, mud therapy is, for sure, a boon for skin rejuvenation.

**Mud Therapy: Two Way Treatment**

Mud Therapy is exercised in two ways

1 Mud Pack

2 Mud Bath

Mud Pack

The mud pack is prepared by taking clay from below the surface of earth. The earth is dug about ten centimeters below ensuring that it should be free from any composite or impurities such as pebbles or decaying matter in the clay. Then the mud practitioner mix warm water with it and prepare smooth paste.

When the paste is cooled down, it is spread on a cloth. Then the mud pack is ready for use. The size of the cloth depends upon your requirement i.e. which part of the body you want to cover with mud pack for treatment. In mud pack, the entire body is not covered, only the effective part is covered.

Needless to say, that several doctors across globe prescribe mud pack to treat diseases relating to nervous disorders and general weakness. Apart from it, by applying mud pack, one can treat fever, influenza, measles, swelling, rheumatism, stomach and ear troubles, kidney problems, liver malfunction, diphtheria, sexual disorder, headache, toothache and general pains in any part of the body.

The cooling effects of mud pack for fever is miraculous. Within minutes, this pack brings down the fever. If mud is applied to the abdomen, the ailment of indigestion, intestinal obstructions, colitis, amoebiasis and flatulence is eliminated. The mud pack is removed after 15-30 minutes depending on its result on different bodies.

Doctors suggest that the affected part should be covered with flannel which is considered a good protective material. Mud pack is also helpful in bacterial diseases. Doctors also suggest that the mode of mud pack treatment should be adopted along with proper dietary system. As the mud retains moisture for a longer period that is the most important benefit of mud pack.

## Mud Bath

In mud bath, people cover themselves directly with the clay. Many people frolic in mud puddles in groups to get the maximum enjoyment and benefit out of a mud bath. In another way, the paste of the clay is spread on a huge cloth. The cloth is then wrapped around the full body. After that the body is covered with one or two blankets. It is a quite different exercise from mud pack. After some time, one can have a cleansing bath with hot water and then a cold water shower to have a fantastic result.

Doctors also dub it a mud massage. After half an hour or more, when the massage is absolutely dried up, it is washed off with clean water but doctors suggest only washing with clean water may not be effective. One should enjoy full shower bath to yield better results- first take bath with warm water then shower bath with cold water.

Mud bath helps in toning up the skin. It energizes the skin tissues. It improves the blood circulation. Mud massage or bath gives instant relief from pains caused by injuries or accidents. Mud baths are generally considered very important for natural beauty treatment. In mud bath, caution is paramount otherwise one might catch cold. Needless to say that these baths are very beneficial as they cheer up the body from within.

They give cool and relaxing experiences. In middle class families, ladies generally don't have mud bath but they, in most cases, use multani mitti (which is known best for its cleansing properties) mixing with rose water for face glow treatment. Its paste is also used for pimples' eradication. After 20-30 minutes, the face is washed off with cleansing water. It is also a kind of mud therapy. If you have the itchy feelings with mud bath, you can have the mud pack or multani mitti experience.

In rheumatic pain, mud bath also helps the patients. Doctors generally advise that duration of mud bath should be approximately twenty to thirty minutes. Like mud pack, this bath is also helpful in relieving chronicle pains and intestinal cramps.

Mud therapy is done by mixing cold water by treating the inflammatory conditions. Although the mud therapy is good for relieving pain of the body and it recovers the lost youth but be cautious, it is not an effective treatment if you are suffering from acute diseases.

## Safest Therapy

Undoubtedly, mud therapy is the safest of all therapies. It doesn't have any kind of side effect. Generally, it is exercised by the mud therapists. If any naturopath applies mud therapy in his treatment, you need not to be afraid because mud has on side effects on the body. Mud therapy is overall a safe exercise. Some people may be allergic to mud. So, you may ask the therapist to make patch test before its proper use on your entire body.

## Other Mud Treatment

Apart from popular mud pack and mud bath, there are several other mud relating therapies which are also useful in retaining youth, freshness in the skin and beauty.

## Peat Therapy

Peat therapy- a kind of mud treatment is also helpful in retaining youth and beauty of the skin. It is also a good treatment for several diseases such as insomnia, arthritis, infertility, muscle and skeleton pain, detoxification, stimulation of immune system etc.

In peat therapy, the mud contains fulvic acids, sulfur, humic, cellulose excepting essential pure water. Peat therapy is applied both in hot and cold pack. This therapy can be applied at house as well as spas. In this therapy, either hot or cold water can be added as per the choice of the patient.

## Peloid Therapy

This therapy is better than peat therapy but it can be performed only in mud treatment spas. Moreover, it is expensive as the mud used in this therapy consists of virgin clay, minerals and humus etc. It's best known for skin diseases, osteoarthritis, rheumatoid, gynecological as well as common health problems. It is a boon for blemishes, wrinkles and blackheads etc.

## Mud Relating Packs

Apart from therapy, mud relating packs also help in skin problems and other health relating disorders etc. Parafango packs are known for helping in the degradation of the collagen and elastane in the skin. It soothes the muscle as well as reduces swelling around the joints.

In these packs, volcanic mineral ash, paraffin and extract of seaweed are contained which is wondrous ingredients for the body, skin and mind of the human beings. There is another popular mud treatment pack- mud mask which is also easily available in the market at any beauty store or chemist shop.

The side effect of mud mask is that they contains dyes and perfumes in it which may cause allergic reactions if you have a sensitive skin. So, you must make the patch test before its proper use on your skin.

For Therapy: Technique to Prepare Mud

In mud therapy, the mud for treatment should be without any type of contaminations. It should be totally free from small stones, grass particles and other impurities. It should be taken from 3-4 feet depth of the surface of the ground. Mud therapists advise that the black mud near the pond is good for therapy. To make the mud clean, it should be dried, powered and sieved to remove all kinds of tiny stones, grass particles or other impurities.

The second important point is: knead the mud adding water in right quantity to make the mud smooth for use. It should neither be tight nor containing too much of water.

Benefits of Mud Therapy

It improve acne repair as well as prevention

It promotes youthful complexion

It has an anti-inflammatory effect

It has anti-aging effect

It helps in regenerating the skin

It helps in easing the muscle tension

It helps in improving blood circulation

It has an exfoliating effect

It soothes arthritis joints pains

It gets rid of dead skin and refines the skin structure

It provides relaxation to the eyes

It gets rid of numerous allergies

It tends to retain water for longer time

It helps in general weakness and nervous disorder

It is helpful for patients suffering from gout, diabetes and glaucoma etc.

Be Connected with Mud to Stay Healthy

Walk barefooted on dry mud for sometime regularly. This exercise will stimulate the acupressure points of the soles boosting the body's defences.

Enjoy the sleep on earth to replenish your energy level. This way, you may heal your body and mind through positive vibrations and electromagnetic forces of our planets.

**Know the Healing Properties of Mud**

The mud is rich in minerals. It has unique healing properties. It is soothing and cooling by nature. It is also used for cosmetic and medicinal purposes since ancient times. It has natural anti toxin and magnetic properties.

That is why in some part of India a peculiar form of mud treatment is practised. The patient is buried in earth up to his neck for fixed hours regularly until he cures properly. Mahatma Gandhi too used mud pack to get rid of constipation. The effects of mud are vital, revitalizing and invigorating. In several cases, we apply the mud bandage on the wound of our body.

Thus, the mud therapy is undoubtedly a natural treatment for the good health of human beings.

## Chapter Eight

## Right Soap for Skin

Most of us often confuse while choosing the right soap for our skin. If you are one of them, this article will help you pick the right type of soap for you. Certainly, most bathing soaps contain some detergents which strip away the skin's natural protective oils which are essentially helpful in retaining the moisture in the skin. Although most soap manufacturing companies claim their products as being gentle yet actually all so-called good soap products are not for all type skins.

## History Beckons

Soap is known as one of the oldest industrial products. If we look back, it was first developed in Roman Times. The types of soap available currently date back seventh century. Today, all soaps are the same in chemical terms as they were in previous centuries except for the difference and growth in its colour and fragrance.

## Know the Nature of Your Skin

Initially, you must know the nature of your skin then determine the type of soap right for you. Most ladies prefer costly fragranced soaps to make their shower delightful.

They don't pay much heed towards the basic attributes of the soap while cleansing the skin especially the soft skin of face. Soap is generally scented with fragrance and essential oils. Essential oils are directly derived from plants while fragrance oils are synthetically created, such combination is not good for the skin. Dermatologists advise that don't run after advertisements and opt for only fragranced soap. Choose the real soap matching to your skin requirements. Your soap must provide natural suppleness to your skin. It is best if you pick natural soap containing antioxidants which will help you protect the skin from pollution.

## Major Types of Skin and Right Soap

There are five major types of skin. Each skin needs different types of soaps.

## Herbal Soap for Normal Skin

Normal skin looks healthy. There is perfect balance between oil and moisture contents in the skin. It is without spots and blemishes.

It appears smooth, clear and toned reflecting good health. Moisturizing and herbal soaps which are natural and ingredients in them are ideal for normal skin.

Such soaps can give best results as these contain the mixtures of vitamins, herbs and natural substances. Such soaps are especially formulated to promote skin health.

## Antibacterial Soap for Oily Skin

Oily skin contains excessive oil which attracts dirt and dust leading to pimples, acnes, black heads, spots etc. It looks greasy. For oily skin, one should try an antibacterial soap. With such types of soaps one can get rid of blemishes, dirt and oil of skin. Antibacterial soap gets rid of toxins from the skin. Moreover, soaps with almond and calendula oils are considered ideal. They are gentle and effective. But such soaps should be used in small amounts.

## Dry Skin and Herbal Soap

Dry skin is not known as good skin type. It always looks parched and flaky. Deficiencies of moisture in the skin lead to its dryness. Its sebaceous glands secrete inadequately to make the skin moistened.

The best soap for this skin is something with oatmeal or avocado extracts. For dry skin, the soap should be made from natural ingredients such as peppermint, lavender or spearmint oils. These ingredients help in getting rid of impurities from the skin.

Dr. Rajesh Parnami advises that the people having dry skin should be alert while shampooing hair. They should keep any shampoo off their face as it can harm their skin depleting its protective lipids.

## Mineral Colorants Soap for Sensitive Skin

Sensitive skin owns fine texture. It is highly sensitive to climatic changes. If one owns sensitive skin, he/she should use the soaps which are made of essential oils.

Dr. Ravindra Lavania opines that soaps with herbal or mineral colorants are good for sensitive skin as these are considered the most natural types and don't irritate the sensitive type skins.

Dr. Lavania further advises that some type soaps generally strip oil from the skin and some people feel irritation on their skins as some ingredients in the soaps are allergic to any particular person with sensitive skin. In such situation, it is better if people with sensitive skin avoid using soaps.

Dr. Anju Sachdeva says that gentle herbs plants viz. chamomile and lavender are ideal for sensitive skin. Moreover, chamomile has a calming effect on the skin. Actually, these herbs work on almost every skin.

Most companies use these herbs when they manufacture soaps for all skins. Without drying, it gets rid of the impurities of the skin. Lavender has some of the same properties. It even promotes sound sleep, Dr. Anju concludes.

## Organic Soap for Combination Skin

In this type of skin, the cheeks and the area around the mouth looks dry. Forehead, nose and chin- known as central panel of the body appear oily. Thus, it is called the combination skin. For this skin, organic soap or soaps having the combination of natural ingredients- oils, flower extracts are ideal.

Organic bath soaps have natural sweet fragrances of lavender, rose, lemongrass etc. Moreover, they do never irritate the skin rather provide some extra benefits. They serve to nourish and rejuvenate the skin.

## How to Determine the Type of Skin

Some ladies are generally unaware how to know the type of their skin. Dermatologist Rajesh Parnami suggests that the pragmatic way to recognize the skin type is to check the level of oil on your face in the morning. He says when you wake up in the morning; wipe your face with hankie or any other tissue.

If you find some oil on your hankie or the tissue paper, then your skin is oily type. If you observe the oil only on your T-Zone Area i.e. forehead, nose and chin then it is combination type.

If you don't find any grease or oil on your hankie or tissue paper, then your skin may be either normal or dry type skin. Dry skin is too tight and parched. Normal skin is supple, smooth and flexible. It is natural way to determine the type of your skin.

## Dermatologist's Opinion

Dermatologist Dr. Mohit Sharma opines that soaps which contain moisturizers such as glycerin or lanolin or fat or oils (coconut or palm) are considered good types. They enable the soap which could cleanse the skin properly. Salt is good antiseptic and is used in good quality soaps.

He further says that most of the normal cheap soaps in the markets are alkaline. They react with the acidity of the skin and decay superficial cells. Its putrefaction causes bad odour. Don't buy cheap soaps. They consist of more alkaline giving more damage to the skin. He suggests that one should buy soaps which are having natural ingredients.

## Natural Soap for All Ladies

Dr. Amit Sachdeva says that the all ladies should buy natural soaps which contain anti oxidants. They will help you protect your skin from the ravages of pollutions and the effects of sun's rays. Such soaps are good to protect your skin from wrinkles.

He further says that each good soap should have performed three functions, one- it should remove surface grime; two, it should cleanse the skin without disturbing the normal balance, three, it should keep the surface of the skin free from dead cells. Body natural soap and glycerin soap have been known for good results.

## Don't Use Any Soap Repeatedly

Chemically, every soap; either they are costly or cheaper- they all are a salt of fatty acids. They are generally made of sodium which is disruptive for the upper layer of the skin. Most dermatologists advise us that we should not use the soap repeatedly because sodium in the product will dry the skin promptly.

Although, most companies have switched to vegetable sources for their brand which give the soap slightly a creamier touch, yet one can't ignore the side effects of its repeated use due to sodium components. Dr. Amit Sachdeva says that some-soaps are nicer to look and shop keepers speak about only their benefits. You must read the ingredients published on the pack before its use. If you need to use the soap repeatedly, try on lotion instead. Some lotions themselves have soap but they don't harm as the soaps.

## All Herbal Soaps Are Good For All Skin?

Dr. Sunir Thakkar says that it is a popular myth that all herbal soaps are good for all skins. Don't believe in it. Some of the herbal soaps cause skin rashes, allergic reactions and give internal damage to the respiratory system.

It all depends on the condition and sensitivity of your skin. If one thinks that he may be allergic to certain plants, he/she must test the soap on the small part of the skin before its regular use for all skin. All herbal soaps are not for all people.

## Use Non Drying Cleanser for Face Washing

Dr. Ravindra Lavania advises that despite the companies claim their product healthy for face skin, both sensitive and oily skin ladies/gents should instead look for gentle non-drying cleansers for the protection of their face. Cleansers generally won't strip away the natural oils of the skin and develop your face dry and tight.

Dr. Lavania further says that in some cases, non dry cleansers are not helpful where face needs aggressive cleansing then you should not use the same soap for your face as you use for your body. Remember, facial soaps are specially designed for sensitive facial skin. Even the mildest body soap is too hard on the face. If you need for soap for acne treatment, buy soap cakes which include salicylic acid and benzoyl peroxide. These are two of the top ingredients which are known as best for acne treatment.

## Chapter Nine

## Protect Your Hair

Generally, women are worried over the fall and breakage of their hair due to choosing wrong cleansing products. They often complain that while combing their hair they look their hair unexpectedly smashed and fell down afterward.

The pertinent question is: are the only wrong cleansing products responsible for the hair damage? In several cases, wrong type of the hairbrush is more responsible than the cleansing products for the damage of their hair.

### For Healthy and Good Looking Hair

Dermatologist Dr. Ashok Parnami says that regular brushing with the right type of hairbrush is essential to keep the hair in healthy and good looking. Brushing itself stimulates the glands in the scalp to distribute oils. So, Dr. Parnami further advises that "for conditioning as well as styling, the hairbrush is indispensable for both men and women of all ages to ensure excellent results".

Beautician Rajni Wadhwa opines that good hairbrushes are an investment for the health of the hair but generally in mediocre families, women are quite casual regarding the choice of right hairbrush to match the type of their hair. They usually underrate the hairbrushes and pick the one which is available in the market.

Always remember, the wrong type of hairbrush will damage not only of your hair but it will ruin your look also, Ms Rajni concludes. Moreover, with the right type of brush, you can not only make your hair look healthier and shinier but you can also achieve the desired look of your face. Right hairbrushes massage the scalp and spread the oil in the scalp.

## When Your Hairs Are Wet

When your hairs are wet, you ought to be more careful because wet hairs are fragile and they moreover require gentle handling. To brush your wet hair, you prefer natural bristle brush than a synthetic one because synthetic materials might cut your fragile and stretched hair.

If you prefer to use comb than hairbrush, choose a wide tooted comb to keep your hair away from any injury. Brushing is very important for both long and short hair. A proper brushing provides the natural oils to the roots of the hair and it also increases the circulation to the scalp and stimulates hair growth.

## How to Brush Your Hair

Beautician Rajni Wadhwa says that brushing the hair itself is an art. For the protection of your hair, you need to remove the large tangle gently with your fingers before using hairbrush then start to brushing and picking up more hair until you reach the scalp.

Then, you do brushing thoroughly from the scalp to the ends with long strokes continuously. Beautician Indu Bala suggests that ladies should brush the hair down toward the floor by bending towards their waist. It is a good exercise as well as method to increase the blood flow which will stimulate the scalp to absorb natural hair oils.

## Match Brush with Your Hair Type

Every hairbrush is not good for everybody. Choose the correct type and size matching to your hair type. If you have thick and coarse hair, you can just pick a paddle brush to make your look smooth and stylish.

Its natural bristles are good to spread the natural hair oils equally as well as it is an excellent way to massage the scalp. If you have medium length hair in a straight cut, cushion style brush is moderate for you because of its flat back designs.

For curly hair, you can choose a round vented brush with rounded ball tips that are shaped as the part of the bristles. Generally, the ball tips are easily broken within short period of its use.

Don't use such hairbrushes which are without nylon ball tips on their bristles. They may cause breakage or damage your curly hair. Curly hairs may be frizzy at times when they are dry brushed. For such hair, toothcomb can be sufficiently helpful.

If you have long hair you should choose preferably a wide toothed comb. Then you can use a vented or round brush. It is best to detangle hair. For straight hair, thermal brush is known best in its use and such brushes are available in flat styles in the markets but they should be used carefully. Ms. Rajni Wadhwa advises that one should always use such hair brushes which are made of natural bristles. Such brushes help stimulate the scalp and nourish the hair follicles. She finally says that if you have fine hair, a vented brush can help you achieve a great look and style.

## Chapter Ten

## Diet: Before and After Work Out

Most of us generally think that exercise with empty stomach helps in losing weight. Is it right? If you think so, you are in the wrong. Exercise with empty stomach or full stomach either is harmful to the body. USA based sports nutritionist Leslie Bonci says that our body needs fuel before exercising in the morning because all the night we have had nothing to eat so before at least half an hour we start the exercise we should take something that is easily digested.

Health Experts say if you want to workout for an hour, you need at least 100 to 200 calories before the start of the exercise which we can get from carbohydrates, protein and fat. People generally go straight to their workplace after their morning exercise without eating something. They normally think eating after the sweat-out negates its effect.

Sanjeev Marshal, a coach at Power House dubs it a wrong myth. If you don't eat something after the morning exercise, you won't refuel your body either way. By eating something, you must compensate the immense energy loss you have done during workout schedule. If you are careless about taking proper food your blood sugar certainly will drop. If you eat after the exercise, you will be able to feed your brain which controls our muscles and mood.

If you are trying to lose weight essentially you must eat something so as you can give your body the energy.

Without energy you will be unable to do exercise but don't take high protein foods like cashew nuts, high fat or sugary foods because they take much time to digest. Moreover, fatty food gives extra calories which hampers in losing weight. Exercise at any time is always good, if you like exercise at gym, you must hit the gym at least thrice a week but you must not feel your stomach heavy at the time of work-out.

After 40-60 minutes exercise or brisk walk, you must take full meal at least one hour after the exercise including pulses, wheat bran, soya; brown rice etc avoiding fatty or sugary food at all.

During exercise, one loses sodium and electrolytes, fruit juice and water can also help you regaining energy. If you are not used to heavy morning breakfast after the exercise, liquids can also supplement you. Before or during exercise, don't forget gulping sufficient water.

Dr. Arun Makker, MD says that five to six moderate meals throughout the day are better than two to three heavy meals. Our body needs sustained energy throughout the day. If you have long gap between your take-in schedules, you can give harm to your body.

If you are long travelling and unable to take meals at proper time, you must carry a bottle of water with you to keep yourself well hydrated protecting from hypoglycaemia. Eat fresh fruits and drink juice during journey to recover your fatigue. Appetite and dehydration causes severe headache and abdomen problem.

Mahesh Bala, physical instructor at Sacred Heart Convent School says that there are several researches suggesting that after exercise simple carbs helps the body in recovering itself quickly so once you are back at home after exercise either morning or evening, you must sit for a small, satisfying feast.

Mahesh Bala next says generally a person having 100-120 pounds burn approximately 80-100 calories after walking a mile. If you have extra weight, walk briskly or on rocky terrain to seek quick, better results.

To ascertain the amount of fluid take-in during workout, you can weigh yourself before exercise. Then after an hour vigorous workout, weigh yourself again without weighing the sweat inside your clothes. Next, replenish your body the fluids recover its loss.

Sanjeev Marshal finally says that he sees several men sweating out on treadmill, simultaneously eating low carb meals also but they remain failed in losing kilo or even an inch. Why? The reason they people are unable to manage their meals before and after their workout properly. The most important point is: manage your meals before and after the exercise, nothing else.

## Chapter Eleven

### Health Dilemma for "Forty Plus"

Are you forty plus? Have you ever thought about the changes in your body? It is the age when we begin to slow down gradually. Forty is, in fact, an important signpost for human body when hormonal changes start influencing our bodies. It is the time to make ourselves alert & conscious. Before, we could fall into health dilemma, it is better to make amends for the resolutions we have inadvertently or carelessly broken the years.

Doctors say that the basal metabolic rate (BMR) - which is particularly helpful in burning calories and keeping the body's several functions in operation such as breathing, cell growth & repair, the rate of heart beating etc. begins to slow down by five percent on average every decade after forty years of age.

Nagpur based Dr. Ravindra Lavania opines that when you are below forty, you enjoy the freedom of eating whatever you binge on. Twenty or thirty is the age of freedom from all anxieties, stress and family responsibilities. At this age, we generally have to work harder and long time. Dr. Lavania further states that, you are then free to crunch potato chips or devour maggi food but after forty, the level of BMR lowers down and it doesn't allow you to eat profusely.

If you are then a bit careless regarding your diet or health, you will gain some extra pounds inviting several health problems. Then the solution is: only physical exercise or regularly brisk walking plus the control on your calories. It might be helpful for you to cut down some extra pounds. Moreover, before forty, one has to have less family related stress and tension. It is the stress & anxiety which invite ailments, Dr. Lavania concludes.

Dr. Anju Setia too says that at forty or above, generally our responsibilities towards our jobs or about the career of our children increase. Several times, due to this, we have to undergo unwanted strain & anxiety. All this increases our bad cholesterol and lower down the good cholesterol in our body and we become the victim of no more than our own lifestyles, Dr. Anju adds.

Dr. Madhu Sharma, a gynecologist says that it is the critical phase of intense hormonal changes in most women because at the age of 40-45 most women begin to hit menopause. Some ladies of this age group begin to eat double the amount as they ate earlier due to lack of essential nutrients in their bodies. Dr. Madhu Sharma next says that at this age, men too begin to experience nutrient deficiencies.

Slowing of the BMR is genetically natural. It happens as the age grows. Also, we can't shirk our job & family responsibilities in this period as well. Then, how we can control our BMR? Dr. Sharma confidently says that check on diet i.e. trim your calories plus doing exercise daily is the best option of keeping the bad cholesterol in check. Dr. Rishu Setia opines that as we age, our metabolism decelerates. Its simple meaning is we begin to burn fewer calories as we burned in our younger days. The simple formula to lose weight is: take fewer calories than you burn, nothing else. When we fail to regulate slowing metabolism, we gain weight.

Sanjeev Marshal, a coach at Power House opines that exercise for "plus-forty" people is one of the most key components to loose weight. Although, exercises have numerous benefits for the people of all ages but the benefits for "plus forty" are even greater. As we grow old, we lose muscle mass and it slows down our metabolism.

Exercises at gym not only help the people strengthening their muscles but they accelerate the metabolism in their body burning more calories. He further advises that a regular routine of 35 to 50 minutes exercise, three to four days a week can help much in keeping off the extra pounds. It is better for both overweight men & women to lose their weight to minimize the health risks. When the body tends to stack excess fat around our mid section; the risk for heart diseases and diabetes increases.

## Diet Advice for "Plus Forty"

Most doctors advise that "plus forty" people must include flaxseeds- which have anti-ageing, anti-inflammatory & estrogenic properties; in their diets. Flaxseeds are helpful in treating arthritis, heart diseases and high blood pressure. Its estrogenic properties help the post menopausal women treating their brittle bones. Flaxseeds are also rich in vitamin B-complex & Vitamin E. Women can take it with water, curd or milk.

Dr. Lavania says that with the growing age, the damage to joints is essential. It is genetic. None can stop it but you can delay it if you frequently use garlic and fenugreek seed. These help in arthritis treatment. Fenugreek is significantly helpful for diabetics, Dr. Lavania adds.

Shimla based Dr. Amit Sachdeva advises that plus forty people must take a teaspoon honey regularly to improve the level of their BMR. Plus, they must eat foods rich in vitamin C such as lemon, oranges and amla. Vitamin C delays wrinkles & makes the skin young-look. It makes our digestive system strong & healthy.  For anti-oxidants, you can eat tomatoes, brinjals, black grapes & carrots etc. Dr. Amit says that anti-oxidants are essential and important for all people but for those plus forty, they are much better.

Dr. Anju Setia advises that plus forty people must take soybeans, milk, pulses & oat also in sufficient quantity. Oat helps in digestion and reduces the cholesterol in our bodies. Soybeans help in protecting against arthritis. After menopause, the bones of women generally become week. Pulses, milk and other foods rich in calcium can help them recover their weakness. For bone health, vitamin D- just an exposure of ten to twenty minutes to sun is enough, Dr. Anju Setia concludes.

## Essential Health Tips for "Plus Forty" Ladies

Although the life of today's women is very hectic & busy yet they are health conscious. Due to their busy work routine, they hardly find any time for physical work. In old days, their life had been quite different. Then the most women did hard physical work routinely and they needed not to do some extra exercise to lose weight. But present scenario is quite different. Here are some most essential health tips for ladies above forty. To remain healthy and fit forever, they should repeatedly read these tips.

Never let your body gain weight. Balance your diet. Burn your calories to poise your body.

Do weight losing activity or exercise regularly. It will keep the heart attack at bay.

Always supplement calcium to your body to make your bones strong.

Quit smoking if you are used to it. Smoking is harmful for both men & women. But it is more harmful for women. It invites several types of cancer apart from heart diseases and lung diseases.

**Never eat oily and spicy food excessively.**

Make a routine for cycling, swimming & aerobic exercises in your life also.

Visit your gynecologist regularly. Contact your family doctor from time to time.

Eat fruits & vegetables sufficiently to get over mood swings and hormonal imbalances. It is common to gain weight before, during and after menopause, so take care in eating healthy food rich in vitamins and minerals.

## Chapter Twelve

### Make Your Smile *Dimpled*

In recent times, the dimply smiles of Preity Zinta, Shahrukh Khan, John Abraham and Arjun Rampal have fascinated greatly both the guys and girls of the country. Everybody wants to attract others by their amazing smiles and thinks of making dimples on their cheeks like them. Certainly, the dimples on the cheeks give the guys and gals a cute and dashing look and make their smiles incredible. It is a craze not only among women but the men of every age are also going in for facial surgeries to have a wonderful smile to magnetize others.

Luckily, some people are naturally adorned with dimples on their cheeks and they are loved by all thanks to their dashing and ravishing smile. Doctors say that dimples are ephemeral; they don't stay forever if one doesn't care about them. Thanks to advancement in cosmetic procedures, in recent times, one can have ravishing dimples on their cheeks with simple procedures just spending Rs: 8000-10000 for single dimple.

### Craze for Creating Dimples

Fashion connoisseurs say that dimply cheeks are mania among youths living in modern society who dream of having movie stars' smile and looks. Dr. Ramesh Gupta, surgeon says that these days, several men are approaching to plastic surgeons to get carried out cosmetic surgery on their cheeks to create lovely dimples like Bollywood stars.

Dr. Ramesh Gupta further opines that not only the youngsters and girls but even the older people are also craving to have looks like film actors. Even engaged and committed girls and boys too are interested to construct a lovely dimple to catch the attention of their partners.

Five years earlier, this craze had been among only young girls but now days, men too have started to visit cosmetic surgeons to have dimple creation surgeries. Also, it is more popular trend among male models working in advertising industry. They think that if they shift to Mumbai in near future, the dimples on their cheeks might help them launching a new career in Bollywood because of the generations' craze for dimpled cheeks or face.

## How Dimples Are Created

Dr. Anju Sachdeva says that dimple is actually a defect on the face due to improper growth of the cheeks muscles. They are caused by having shorter muscles in certain areas of the face. Generally, dimples are genetically inherited and are dominant traits. A rarer form is the single dimple, which occurs on one side of the face only. We generally see that younger babies have dimples but sometime later, they disappear or become less noticeable because with the increase in age, muscles too lengthen.

Dr. Anju further says that if the muscles are not fully developed, a slight serration is observed which makes the smile cuter than normal faces without the serration. So, to create an artificial dimple on cheeks is simple. It is in fact an artificial process which simulates a serration on the face.

In this method, a punch biopsy instrument is placed against the inner cheek and circular motions are made to cut the fat and cheeks muscles leaving the skin intact which create a shallow cylindrical shaped defect under the skin. Then, the doctor closes this defect by doing absorbable stitches to the cheek muscle or through the dermis layer of the skin. Finally, a surgical knot is tied which results in dimpling of the skin even without smiling.

## Surgery and Laser Methods

Dr. Anju Sachdeva next says that there are two procedures to create dimples on face- surgery and laser. In surgery, fat is removed from inside and cheeks are stitched. This surgical procedure takes just half an hour for one cheek. If your cheeks are chubby, to remove the bigger core of soft tissue, the doctor will use a bigger punch biopsy to see better results. If one is interested to have a dimple on both cheeks, he/she has to spend less than one hour with the cost of maximum 18000-20000.

Surgical technique involves simulating the natural way a dimple is constructed by connecting the skin and the cheek muscle. With surgery, the muscle contracts pulling the skin inward side creating a dimple. The other method of constructing the dimple is laser technology. In this method, after anesthesia, the fat is burnt from inside. In recent times, laser is known as the better way to create dimples because there is less pain and less bleeding. Doctors say that skin takes a week or two to flatten out when the suture is absorbed.

## Essentially After Care

After the dimple simulating process; patient notices minimal swelling and pain and doctors prescribe the patient some painkiller medicine and antiseptic solution plus antibiotic intake. But in the ecstasy of having amazing dimply smile you don't forget to have the intake of medicine in time. After the surgical process, regular mouth rinsing with an antiseptic solution is must. Normally, the patient heals in four days but it takes minimum 14 days for the dimple to be seen. Don't forget to rinse the mouth meanwhile to have a better result of your dimple appearance.

## Chapter Thirteen

## BEAUTY AND GOOD LOOKS

## IN THE HANDS OF COSMETOLOGIST

Beauty lies in the eyes of beholders? Today, is it true? Undoubtedly, it's an excellent saying and moreover a sample of poetic universal reality - but in our day, in actuality, with the changed fashion world, it might not be an exaggeration if one says that beauty lies in the salon of cosmetologist or in the hands of those experts who have made it their business to make others' look attractive, gorgeous, pleasing and more importantly impressive, sweet and charming.

### Don't Shy of Visiting Saloons

Beautician Rajni Wadhwa says that beauty and good looks play an important role in enhancing the personality of ladies. Beauty attracts everybody. It is also necessary for professional growth. Needless to say, beautiful ladies get more salary than those of plain ladies.

Gone are the days when people shy of visiting the beauty saloons. Cosmetic counseling which is also known as anti ageing counseling is at present becoming popular day by day and beauty conscious ladies, with the modern times, are flocking to cosmetic surgery clinics for tummy tucks, face lift, hair removal, dimpled or sculpted smiles and parrot like sharp noses etc.

Rajni Wadhwa further says that, for sure, beauty lies in the eyes of beholders but at present, the scalpel of a cosmetic surgeon has sharpened enough to enhance the beauty of any lady or a gentle man. After the surgery, it is the prime duty of a beautician to retain the beauty of her customers forever.

So, the beauty is the business of both the cosmetic surgeon and the beautician. So, don't hesitate visiting beauty saloons regularly while having appointments with your cosmetic surgeon as well for the counseling, Rajni concludes.

## Visit an Expert Cosmetic Surgeon

Present age is an era of hi-tech, state-of-the-scalpel system. It is not the age of b*esan-malai* home made packs. These days, such home made packs are not generally used in hi-fi standard families by reason of not giving amazing and quick results like cosmetic surgery.

That is why; beauty conscious ladies hailing from decent upper strata of society generally prefer to visit beauty saloons for their beauty treatments and therapies in preference to applying home made solutions.

Dr. Anju Sachdeva says that health and beauty are complimentary and interdependent issues. Interaction between and doctors and the beauticians is necessary for the best result in enhancing the physical beauty.

Therefore, ladies! If you are really dreaming of queen like beauty, always visit an expert (who is medically qualified with a thorough knowledge of cosmetology, beauty therapies and the science of human anatomy) for your cosmetic surgery.

Dr. Anju further says that without expertise and know-how, cosmetic surgery can have disastrous complications such as suture problems or like that. Carelessness in beauty treatment ruins your skin resulting in undesirable scars.

So, never think of money if it is the case of your gorgeous beauty and good looks. Don't come to the money in your way if it is the question of facial deformities or body carving treatments.

Beauty Centre these day are offering every treatment from trimming fat, erasing laugh lines to removing excess baggage under the eyes etc. apart from hair, feet, hands and the treatments of every part of the body.

## Why Beauty is Necessary

Needless to say that professional success and fame also depend on how beautiful and fit you look. At present, thanks to media exposure, even politicians and socialite ladies have to concentrate on their looks to attract public attention. In every business, beauty pays more than one expects.

Apart from several high profile professions, profession like receptionists, modeling, acting and PR agencies, an important weightage is also given to one's external personality and good looks. So, ladies! Beauty is necessary for your reputation and respect in the society and for your growth in professional life. When you visit the parlor, beauty specialists will advise you how to discover the type of the skin and how to take care of it in humidity as well as in sunlight.

## Be Careful While Removing Tattoos

At the start, complex designs tattoos attract the ladies enchantingly but after some times, they become the objects of frustration and boredom and they wish to have them removed as early as possible. The removal of tattoos is more difficult and painful than its carving out. If they are removed carelessly by inexperienced cosmetologist, they may result in ugly scars, pigmentation and keloids.

Ladies! If you are planning to have your tattoos removed, never visit a low profile cosmetologist. You may save your money but lose your beauty and health. Always remember that beauty is always more important than money. Removal of tattoos keeps the skilled dermato surgeons always busy.

Fix an appointment with him/her whether you have to wait for several weeks. Don't forget an expert dermato surgeon has refined techniques for skin resurfacing. He/she has the ability to remove tattoos, acne scars and smallpox scars etc. carefully.

## Cosmetic Surgery Techniques

Chemosurgery, laser treatment, micro dermabrasion, photo rejuvenation, electro-depilation, radio surgery, electro-surgery and laser epilation are several names in the history of modern treatments for beauty enhancement programmes. A little scar, mole or mark on the face of any lady is always a cause of anxiety and frustration. It ruins the glow of her face and upset her mood. To get rid of such scars, electro-surgery is known the best modern method for scar/mole disappearance. Moreover, electro surgery also promises to take care of common skin problems like warts and skin tags etc.

Dr. Rajesh Sharma says that some time ago, pumice stone was used to remove facial hair but today, there are several innovative alternatives for the removal of facial hair such as electrodepilation and laser epilation etc.

For skin treatment, radio surgery is equally important and it is also a popular treatment. In this treatment, patients don't feel the burning of surrounding skins despite that there is knife life sharpness in this therapy.

Dr. Amit Sachdeva says that in micro dermabrasion, micro crystals of aluminium are used for the treatment of scars and pigmentation. It is no doubt a success therapy.

Dr. Rohit Lavania says that apart from other body parts, nose is also focused for cosmetic surgery. Several ladies wanted their nose like Bollywood queen Aishwarya Rai and they asked their surgeons to shape it the same.

Dr. Lavania further says that during the wedding season, they have several requests for cosmetic surgeries. Dr. Anju Sachdeva says that now-a-days, the most sought after facial treatment is Botox because it is quick and easy treatment. During wedding seasons, both ladies and gents prefer to take on this treatment.

## Prevention Factor

No doubt, cosmetic expert is able to make you a dashing queen but to retain the earned beauty for longer time; it is your own duty to take some preventive steps. It's truly said that prevention is better than cure.

Dr. Amit Sachdeva says that treatments are okay but if you are failed to have a sound sleep and balanced diets, you won't be able to retain your health and glowing look for longer period.

Balanced diets and sound sleep are essential for a healthy body and glowing looks. Lack of sleep certainly will make you look older than actually you are. It may produce dark circles under your eyes. Thus, always remember that those who binge on junk food and are far away from fruits and green veggies definitely have skin problems.

If one conquers the skin problems with expensive treatments but don't stop junk foods, he/she again has to experience several skin diseases. Nutritionist Rekha Sharma suggests that before making an appointment with a cosmetologist, visit a dietician and make sure you are taking proper diets suitable for your skin type and lifestyle.

A regular brisk walk without a break is better than weekly workout in any gym. Sanjeev Marshal, a gym trainer opines that improper diets make the body deprives of essential nutrients and causes havoc to the skin. Moreover, lack of essential body exercise makes the skin wrinkle and sagging. With the help of dermatologist, undoubtedly, you may improve your health but it would be for the time being. To look and feel better for a long time, you have to work hard and love yourself.

## Facial Massage for Skin Glow

Apart from surgery, cosmetologists and beauty consultants generally believe that regular massage is an essential exercise to check further aging or at least it slow down the ageing process. Noted facial massage therapist Belle Tuckerman opines that massage is a great stress reducer as it gives the wonderful relaxation experience. It is certainly an antidote to ageing.

Rajni Wadhwa, a beautician says that the benefits of massage are much more than that our eyes see. Our skin has two distinct layers. The first layer is known as epidermis which itself consists of six layers. The ageing process transpires with these layers. When dead skin cells begin to surface, they make the skin looked aged.

To make the skin fresh, new and bright, new cells are needed to replace the dead cells and it only can happen by doing vigorous massage. Vigorous massage is known as skin rejuvenation therapy. Under the epidermis lies the dermis – a second layer of skin which is comparatively deeper. It is the place where sweat and oil glands, blood vessels, hair follicles, nerves and muscle tissues are positioned.

Moreover, human body's chief support structure- collagen is also situated in dermis. A break down in collagen- the body structure is the cause of wrinkles and crinkles. It is the only reason of sagging skin.

## Who is Cosmetologist?

A cosmetologist is a trained professional possessing the understanding and perception of aesthetics. He/she is well versed in styling techniques and aware of contemporary beauty fashions. He/she is an integral part of the beauty business and beauty saloon industry. He/she is known as beauty specialist who is well educated in treating the hair, skin and nails etc.

The skilled hands of a cosmetologist may make the ladies the queen of the event or any festival they desire. A cosmetologist is one who performs manicures, haircutting, styling, makeup, facials, hair and scalp treatments, head and neck massages and full body care, shampooing etc. Moreover, a cosmetologist also advises on use of right type cosmetics, skin, care lotions and makeup application etc.

Needless to say that a cosmetologist renders personalized beauty care from head to toe. He/she chooses cosmetics that are apt for client colouring and his/her skin tone. He/she is able to shape, trim, pluck and colour the eyebrows also. In the treatment of nails, he/she cleans the fingernails or toenails, treat cuticles.

A flattering hairstyle and the right touch of makeup by an expert cosmetologist can play up your best features to draw attention of others towards you.

In general, cosmetologists are self employed. They have their beauty saloons. In some cases, they are also employed in beauty saloons, spas, cosmetic departments or barber shops run by several other businessmen.

## Chapter Fourteen

### Music Therapy

Music plays a vital role in our life. Its' advantageous, amazing and miraculous effects on the body and the mind in many powerful ways have proven. Needless to say, music helps ward off stress, anxiety and depression. That is why, in recent times, in almost all prominent hospitals, music therapy is used apart from medication

If you are feeling pain in your body and constantly getting your blood pressure high and then in spite of writing a new prescription, your doctor reduces the quantity of your pre-prescribed dose and advises you to buy an IPod or music system, don't laugh at him. He is quite right and knows the therapeutic treatment of music which works more than medicines in most cases.

Several medical researches show that slow paced music can calm the nerves and control blood pressure by inducing endorphins. So, the doctors in general use music as remedial tool.

Why don't you make the music as a routine of your life and listen to your favourite music in your leisure time to keep yourself fit, happy and healthy, but don't forget that fast music or high musical crescendo may give you worse effects instead.

If you are not in a lovely mood then it may increase your blood pressure by causing the blood vessels under the skin to narrow but for relaxation, slow paced music is a proven treatment.

## Music beats stress

Continuing stress wreaks havoc on our cardiovascular system. It may cause our blood vessels to harden constricting the flow of the blood. As the age increases, hardening of the arteries becomes an undying problem. Due to constricted vessels, the level of blood pressure also remains high and it increases the risk of heart attack and stroke.

Continuing stress suppresses the immune system which later becomes the reasons of infertility or impotence apart from speeding up of the ageing process.  But music has the power to counter the effects of stress.

It has long been established that music beats stress and reduces tension. It helps the body not to produce stress hormone known as "cortisol" which causes the body to be strained, not relaxing it a bit to heal and to restore. Less cortisol means lower blood pressure and sound sleep.

If you are a patient of insomnia and used to pills before you go to bed, stop it for some time and listen to slow, cool and tranquil music then see the result. It will check cortisol setting off a positive spiral on your stress syndromes.

After that you may forget the pills and doctor. Chronicle patients should take some medicines with music therapy. If you have no long history of ailment, music therapy alone (without medicines) can help you getting well. Doctors say that calm music is the best treatment to help you having a sound and relaxed sleep.

The use of music by a trained professional has achieved therapeutic goals. Health experts opine that music in conjunction with medicine work wonders. Only medicine take longer time to heal but music definitely reduces the time of treatment.

## Music helps children with speech problem

Also, music works best for all those children who have speech problem. It soothes the nerves as well as stimulates cognitive functioning and correct speech problem. The brain processes music in both the right and the left hemispheres and this process helps children to improve their language or speech.

Don't misunderstand the music as a pure medicine. Only music doesn't really heal. It just pacifies the mind. The combination of the prescribed medicines and listening to soft and calm music regularly give better results.

Music is much better for teenagers or children to improve their memories and concentration than the grown-up. It is the calming and relaxing effects of the music that medico fraternity has begun to motivate people to listen to music as a therapy along with medicine.

## Music recovery is fast

I'm hundred per cent sure that music recovery or therapy is faster treatment than the treatment done by only medicines. Neither only music nor only medicine can alleviate the pain, stress and other mental problems. The conjunction of medicines with music therapy is the best and the quickest treatment.

Several reports reveal that music has some good effects even on the comatose patients. Our body is made up of drones and vibrations; so is the music. And, it reaches the brain through sensory systems. Music stimulates the crucial brain nerves and it gives the positive results.

Always listen to soft and calm music. It is the best as it evokes the finger movements and increases the heart rate as well. Some doctors suggest listening to ragas- Kalyani or Hindola for fast recovery apart from medical treatment.

It has medically proved that ragas give happy expressions. They control the blood pressure of even those patients who are surviving on ventilators. Medical studies show that patients with expressive brain damage and even comatose patients have recovered faster with the combination of music and drugs.

## Music helps the pregnant women

Music therapy is equally useful for pregnant women also. It reduces their psychological stress at the painful time of delivery. More than ninety percent pregnant women had normal labour and had to struggle less during the time of delivery provided you give them a chance to listen to music. Needless to say that the soothing effects of the music do wonders on their nerves and minds.

I strongly advise everybody should listen to music essentially. It might be much better if the pregnant women listen to music for half an hour daily for at least three four weeks during pregnancy to give soothing effects to the unborn baby.

During pregnancy, generally women have nausea and sleep problem due to the increasing size of the fetus. That time, they feel much hard to find a comfortable sleeping position. In such a trouble period, soft and calming music may help pregnant women in feeling delight and comfortable sleep.

## Prominent hospitals start music therapy

A long time ago, North Texas University had announced the music benefits for bed-ridden patients. Recently, the prominent hospitals across India have started to incorporate the use of music in the wards of hospital to help patients for quick recovery.

Music is a wonder treatment because of its resemblance between the patterns of the electrical signals in the brain and that of the musical compositions. The Mayo Clinic in Rochester, Minnesota preferably uses music as part of its cardiovascular surgery healing program to promote relaxation and reduce tension, anxiety etc.

A doctor at Lilavati Hospital, Mumbai had once told me that they play soothing Indian classical and western music in the ICU. For foreign patients, they use Mozart and Beethoven.

It has proved that music either it is the classical or the western music, it helps the patients in recuperating quickly. So, accept the healing power of music and don't forget to buy an IPod and listen to music daily. Don't wait when you are ailing you will listen to the music.

One of my friends, Dr. Pankaj Aneja, PGIMR, Chandigarh would say that listening to music have many positive effects on both the body and the mind But listening to music of every type is not the treatment.

The quickness of healing depends on the interests of the patients which kind of music they like to listen. Generally, in the wards of hospitals, most forms of the music are therapeutic. They play the music on low volume which has soothing healing power. Instead, harsh, loud and discordant music give bad effects on the ailing patients.

## During surgery, music is comfortable

You must have noticed that the surgeons generally play calm, slow and relaxing music during surgical operation. It is because they understand that slow music settles down the patients and they help the doctors to make the surgery a success.

It is a hundred percent proved truth the patients listening to music during and after the operation don't feel as much pain as the patients without music.

## Loud music is not for patients

Fast music is not quite relaxing but if you are not a patient and love to enjoy music for just fun and entertainment; fast music may be wonderful for you also. We see most people feel their pulse go up when they listen to fast and loud music.

Its' constant listening may be bad for the heart if you are somewhat upset but it is sure that it helps you to improve your concentration power. Several medical tests made with people used to loud and fast music has showed that their bodies react in a similar way to fast music as common or ordinary people react to soothing music but fast music is not for patients or the people who want to rest and relax.

## Use music while exercising

Let me suggest you the important points.

When you go for exercise, use the music. Definitely, you will see better results. The beat and sometimes the aggressiveness of the music are helpful when one exercises. In gyms, music is widely used for exercises because it is well known fact it has a good effects on physical activities. Not only it help you during the exercising but it relaxes and heals you post exercise also. After a hard workout, muscles need the rest and it is the calmness of music which relieves and soothes our body.

## Miracles of slow music

- ✓ It keeps the depression and anxiety at bay
- ✓ It lowers the blood pressure
- ✓ It reduces the risk of stroke and heart attack
- ✓ It boosts the immunity
- ✓ It eases the muscle tension
- ✓ It helps you sleep well

✓ It produces the relaxation effects on cardiovascular and respiratory systems.
✓ It always keeps the body young. By listening to music regularly, one can observe the aging process being slowed down.
✓ It improves the mood of the patients and helps them sleep better during recovery.

## How to enjoy the music's delights

For your health and complete well being, let me suggest you some tips to enjoy the music delights in your leisure hours.

1    Take a warm shower before you start to listen to soft and calming music.

2    Listen to your music minimum half an hour daily to relax your strained nerves.

3    During music session, wear loose and comfortable clothes. You can listen to the music by sitting on the chair or lying on the comfortable bed.

4    Turn off the lights and close your eyes when you listen to music.

5    Don't listen to the same tune repeatedly. It diminishes its effects on the body.

6    You can't get that boost if you listen to the same song again and again. One needs to vary the songs each time so when you listen to the new song, it will bring back the sense of delight and happiness.

7    If you are residing in the noisy area. Then use headphones to minimize background noise and get maximum benefits of the music.

## Chapter Fifteen

### Irregular Menstrual Cramps

Menstruation or 'menses' or 'periods' of women is a kind of vaginal bleeding that happen each month. When a woman has her period, she is menstruating. If you are a victim of your hasty lifestyle, or are slapdash in your diet routine or binge on alcohol, junk food etc, none can stop you from suffering from painful menstrual periods. Do you know how to cope with irregular menstrual cramps?

Some times, ladies experience menstrual cramps due to irregularity of their periods. More than one-in-four party going ladies are so badly affected at the time of their periods that they have to take time off from their workplace or school/college etc. Extreme stress, anxiety, unhappiness and lack of insomnia are also some causes of this mess.

### What is menstruation cycle?

Menstruation or 'menses' or 'periods' of women is a kind of necessary vaginal bleeding that happens each month. When a woman has her period, she is menstruating. Menstrual blood is the combination of blood and tissue that drops each month from the lining of the uterus. It flows from the uterus through the small cavity in the cervix and comes out through vagina.

Menstruation is a part of menstrual cycle, which helps the body in preparing for the possibility of pregnancy. The first day of the menstrual cycle is when the bleeding begins to flow out. The average menstrual cycle is almost 28 days long. The rise and fall of body chemical or hormones during the month make the menstrual happen.

## Experiences of menstrual cramps

The sensitivity of the body is quite different in different women. During periods, some ladies feel a transitory uneasiness, while for others it becomes doubled with ache.

Normally, the pain comes in cramp-like spasms, starting off from lower abdomen or lower back and then spreading out to the entire body. Some even suffer from dizziness, fatigue, nausea, vomiting etc.

Period is not the same every month, and also it's not the same as other women's periods. Generally, periods are of three types; long and heavy, short and light and moderate.

Most menstrual periods last from three to five days. They are dubbed as moderate periods. If they stretch to seven days or more, it must be considered quite abnormal.

Periods typically cause women to endure pain for a few hours before its start, which continues for the following days. Generally, pain alleviates when menstrual flow begins. Teenagers undergo more menstrual cramps, while married women sometimes even don't have a bit of feeling about periods.

At the start of menstruation in girls, periods may be very irregular for some months, which become normal gradually with mild treatment. And, they may also become irregular in women approaching menopause.

## Why menstrual pain?

It is the physical condition of women which is responsible for menstrual pain. In some women, the pain results from the passage of menstrual blood through a narrow cervix. During menstrual cycle, in which an egg is released, the pain heightens.

Sometimes, a disease such as uterine fibroids or endometriosis causes the pain. During menstruation, prostaglandins, which are hormone-like substances, are released and causes severe pain in the body.

Prostaglandins serve three primary functions- one, they cause the uterus to contract; second, they reduce blood supply to the uterus, and third, they increase the sensitivity of nerve endings in the uterus to feel the pain.

Such women should take biochemical salts or minerals to cover up their deficiency. They will bring your body back into balance naturally, with no side effects. It's the best formula to treat many physical disorders. But if the pain is intolerably severe, ladies can take any pain killer such as ibuprofen or something like that.

## When to contact a gynecologist

Girls/ladies should contact the gynecologist in such situations.

1. If they have not started menstruating by the age of sixteen
2. If the period of bleeding is more than a week.
3. If their period suddenly stopped.

4. If they have severe pain during the periods
5. If they are bleeding excessively.
6. If they feel sick even after changing the pad.

## How to delight your mood during menses?

During menstrual cycle, the mood is sometimes absolutely upset. To keep your mood happy ands pleasing, change your eating habits to make your mood stable and delightful.

1. During periods, eat fibre-rich diet with lots of fresh fruits and green vegetables.
2. Include pulses, sprouts, soyabean and cereals in your meals.
3. Avoid chocolates, butter, cheese, samosas, ice cream, noodles, pastries etc.
4. If you tend to non-vegetarian, eat only fish. Avoid mutton or chicken.
5. Avoid all forms of sugar viz. sweet, candy, tea etc.
6. No alcohol, no smoking.
7. Drink sufficient water regularly.
8. Do aerobic exercise daily necessarily.
9. Read good, interesting books or magazines.
10. If your abdomen pain is uncontrollable, place a hot water bottle on your abdomen quickly.

## Some other relief tools

1      Hydrotherapy

2      Acupressure

3      Aromatherapy

4        Abdominal Massage

Hydrotherapy is a type of treatment in relieving menstrual cramps through heat. In olden times, elderly women advised young teenagers' and granddaughters to adopt this therapy. Heat increases circulation and reduce muscular tension. So, to get the immediate relief, a hot pack of sand, cloth or water can be placed on the abdomen.

In Acupressure, some certain points are adroitly pressed that are believed to be connected with internal energy pathways to the pelvic area. Through this technique, one can get fully relieved of the pain, if the doer is experienced otherwise this technique would devastate the body with extremely unbearable pain.

The application of oil on the abdomen, hips and lower back is dubbed as Aromatherapy. Many ladies experience uterine cramp relief adopting this method of treatment.

Massage on the abdomen is also another method to increase uterine circulation, thus easing muscular tension. In fact, it's very effective treatment to stop menstrual pain.

## Chapter Sixteen

## Drink Green Tea and Physical Fitness

Several researches reveal that green tea is a healthy beverage. It is being used as a miraculous treatment for a wide range of ailments for more than four thousand years. Thanks to its curative as well as therapeutic powers, it is now labeled as a global brand for health and fitness. Because of its amazing benefits, the level of consumption for green tea has skyrocketed throughout the globe.

You must have heard about the health benefits of green tea. But, if you binge on it, it may ruin your health. A few people know that green tea is totally different from black tea that we drink regularly. If we drink green tea properly and in right quantity daily, it may produce better results. Never drink green tea repeatedly. It may harm your health. However, let me know you the health benefits of Green Tea.

### Health benefits of green tea

- ✓ It is helpful in boosting your vitality. Also, it is an effective way to lose your extra pounds.
- ✓ Green tea contains Egigallocatechin Gallate (EGCG) which includes healing properties. It wipes out cancer cells with no harm to other healthy tissues in the body.
- ✓ EGCG slows down and stops the growth of new cancer cells in the body. All types of cancer- stomach, ovarian, oral, prostate, breast, cervical and cancer of colon- can be cured by drinking green tea.

- ✓ EGCG plays an effective role to stop blood clots formation also which is the main cause of strokes and hearth attacks.
- ✓ EGCG antioxidants in green tea accelerate energy expenditure in the body and stimulates fat metabolism which helps the body not to gain weight.
- ✓ Green tea defends the skin from ultraviolet light radiation.
- ✓ Regular use of green tea makes the teeth and gum tissues healthier apart from other dental benefits.
- ✓ Polyphenols in green tea stops plaque from sticking to the enamel of teeth which reduces the risk of cavity development. Moreover, some green teas contain fluoride which strengths teeth but we should not take it as a replacement for regular brushing and dental care.
- ✓ Green tea checks the growth of bacteria in mouth which cause bad breath.
- ✓ Green tea reduces cholesterol levels.
- ✓ It is a possible cure for obesity.

## If you drink green tea excessively and repeatedly

Green tea is a miracle brew which includes natural ingredients to help the body to be healthy but it is also important to know that there are some negative effects of green tea leaves if you drink it repeatedly more than thrice a day. Remember, some bodies are not compatible for the diet of every type. So, before you have a green tea, think twice and then try just once. Think, is it really right for you. Green tea comes from a bush of Camellia family. This bush is evergreen and shinny that has a wonderful aroma and beautiful flowers. So, green tea is flavorsome.

Because, the green tea is high in caffeine, so the women who are breastfeeding should not excessively drink this tea otherwise they may pass the caffeine on the baby. Nursing women should also avoid taking green tea excessively. I would suggest that even the small amount of green tea powder which is used for baking, smoothies and other foods should be avoided while you are nursing a baby.

**If you are allergic ...**

Green tea is harmful to all those individuals also who are allergic to this beverage. Some people are caffeine sensitive, if they drink green tea regularly, they may develop some rash or hives on his/her body. As caffeine is strong stimulant that can excite the central nervous system resulting the series of ailments such as insomnia, excessive urination etc. If you have already some health problem, before drinking green tea, you must seek the opinion of your doctor.

**If you drink green tea for good health then**

**Remember.....**

1. Brew the tea at the right temperature. The temperature between 56- 62 degree celsius is considered ideal.
2. Drinking scalding hot green tea is damaging to digestive system while cold tea gathers phlegm.
3. Never delay to drink freshly brewed tea otherwise its colour darkens and fragrance evaporates. Through oxidation, tea compounds also lose their potency.

4    Green tea contains amino acids. If you leave it longer, you will find bacteria starts to breed in it. Moreover, vitamins C and B also will diminish over the time.

5    The tea which has been left overnight you don't ever drink. Always drink hot tea.

6    Don't brew tea leaves more than 2-3 grams for a cup to protect you from gastric acids problem.

7    Don't drink over brewed tea. It tastes bitter and is considered harmful for the body.

8    Never take green tea with meal. It is better if you maintain a gap of minimum two hours between meal and tea.

9    Tea can block the absorption of nutrients and harm to your lungs also.

10    Never drink tea if your stomach is empty. Such practice can cause indigestion.

11    Don't drink green tea with medicines or when you are suffering from fever. Green tea can interact with medications, so; as a precaution; avoid tea for at least two hours after taking medications.

12    Some people consume medicine with tea thinking the tea will help them in temperature. Instead, tea increases the body temperature.

13    Never mix your tea with alcohol. It is harmful for kidney, sexual organs and it causes constipation.

## Chapter Seventeen

## Sexual Life and Physical Fitness

Talk on sex in middle-class Indian families is always taboo. Not only the girls, but the guys also are reserved about discussing sex with the sister, mother, aunties or any other female member of the family. It is supposed to be a kind of misdemeanor and idiocy. Do you know the value of sex? It is an energy booster and a dosage for health and fitness

The sex experts opine that sex is one's need to keep the body fit and healthy. It satiates the body's starvation. Having sex with a partner is as good as having a healthy and balanced diet with full of vitamins and proteins.

Many studies show that regular sex is a dosage for health, wellbeing and fitness. It increases the immunity from viruses, relieves stress and anxiety, and moreover, gives delightful relaxation. While making sex, several chemicals emanate from the body which perk up our mood and alleviate the pain of the body. Relaxation after successful sex gives both the partners a kind of pleasure, which help them to recover from the perils of stroke, high blood pressure and depression etc.

Sex helps in protecting the health of man's prostate gland, by emptying the fluids deposited there. So, healthy people should have regular sex to maintain their wellbeing. Some women think that, after menopause, there is an end to sex. "No"- doctors say "menopause doesn't affect one's sexual drive; there is no reason that the healthy men and women shouldn't enjoy their sexual life after menopause.

The intensity of sex may diminish with the ripeness of age but it's the libido satisfaction which makes the body healthy and in the pink. It has nothing to do with the ripened age. Sex can be enjoyed at every age. Due to purported ethics, if you are forced to hold back your sexual desires, you deliberately invite series of ailments.

**Let me tell you some health benefits of sex.**

**Lose your body weight**

It is hundred percent realistic that regular sexual activity is one way to maintain your body healthy and fit. There are about 3500 calories in a pound of fat. If you want to burn these calories, you have to work out for some long hours.

Medical experts say yoga burns 115 calories per half hour. Dancing 130 calories, walking 3 kilometer burns 150 calories, weight training 150 calories and sexual intercourse burns approximately 153 calories per half hour- the maximum burn. If you are one who knows the methods to expand the time of sexual activity, you can burn some more calories.

The more you engage in sexual activities, the more you burn your calories and lose your weight.

**Intensifying blood flow**

Sex intensifies the flow of blood in your brain and other organs of your body. It is one type of exercises, which is even more vigorous than the ground race or brisk walking. It increases both the throbbing of the heart and the breathing rate, which account for the improvement in blood circulation.

As the fresh supply of blood starts, the cells, muscles and organs are flooded with fresh oxygen and hormones. With the circulation of blood, waste products in the body, which cause fatigue and illness too, rapidly eliminate.

## Eradicating stress and anxiety

Sex is the best medicine in handling stress and anxiety. Normal stresses of life don't become the cause of distress for those who enjoy sex frequently.

After satisfyingly lovemaking, when orgasm lets the fatigue go, the freshness of washes down the mess of the heart. After making successful ejaculation, both men and women sleep more deeply and restfully. Even the patients of insomnia can take benefits from sexual pleasure.

## Respite from pain

Medical research says that sex is an amazing pain reliever. It's a remedy for headache, arthritis pain, whiplash pain etc. During sexual activities, arousal and orgasm increases the levels of oxytocin. It spikes the organ 3 to 5 times higher than its usual position before orgasm.

In fact, it is the oxytocin that prompts the orgasm. Oxytocin hormone is secreted in the body which causes the discharge of endorphins, which become the medicine of analgesia and gives respite even from severe pain.

## Always be young hale and hearty

For a long and healthy life, sex is an elixir. A British study shows that those who enjoy sex, at least two times sex a week, have half the death rate as compared to those who indulge in sex less than once a month.

Lack of sexual activities upset the mood and give discomfort. DHEA- a kind of most abundant hormone in the body which secretes during sexual exercise prompts the sexual excitement and increases the response to it.

It helps in balancing the immune system, maintaining and repairing tissues, keeping the skin healthy and supple. It also improves cognition, the cardiovascular system and promotes the growth of bones.

The DHEA hormone is made from cholesterol. The import point is: after it is secreted from adrenal glands, it is changed into whatever hormones the body requires. This system of modification keeps the men and women young, hale and hearty.

## For heart, bones and muscles

Regular sexual activity increases testosterone level in men and estrogen level in women. Testosterone hormones strengthen our bones and muscles also. These keep our hearts healthy and in the pink. It's the only testosterone hormones which compel the men to have a sex and these make women more aggressive.

Women's estrogen hormone makes them more receptive and responsive to men's advances also. These hormones make the woman soft and their breasts taut. Apart from orgasm, these hormones make both women and men hale and hearty and keep their health in peak condition.

## Lower cholesterol

Human body itself makes 80 percent of Cholesterol in the liver. The rest of 20 percent, it gets through eating sugar, fats, proteins etc. When there is too much cholesterol in our body, it tends to stick to the artery walls where it becomes the cause of high blood pressure.

It can lead to blood clots, if there are blockages in the arteries. Blockages in arteries can become the reason of stroke or cardiac arrest, anytime. Regular sex gives us exercise benefits. It helps in lowering the overall cholesterol level, and protects the human beings from severe cardiac arrest.

## Intimacy: a healing power

A research says that the intimacy factor in sex has a healing benefited. No doubt, sex is as good as an exercise, but if love is emotionally involved with it, it is much better. An open heart can lead to most joyful and ecstatic sex, in intimate lovemaking, the risk of premature death and diseases from all cause maybe three to five times less.

The chemical composition of your body can change by a soft and intimate touch. Healthy blood, healthy bones, healthy heart, healthy body and a peaceful mind; all thanks to the healing power of sex.

## Here are some tips to improve the SEX DRIVE

**Healthy diet:** Have a healthy and balanced diet with lettuce, fruits, salads, vegetables and full of proteins. It may reduce your stress, increase your energy and help your body to look and feel better. It is a simple formula of giving and taking. If you give your body a healthy diet, the body will give your energy, mood and strong, amazing sex power.

**Exercise**: Make a routine for physical exercise for at least 20-30 minutes daily. It may improve your energy level. You can exercise or jog, while watching TV, or otherwise, go for a brisk walk. Do whatever you want, but remember your body must feel activated and energized. If you are happy with your body, you body will be happier and will tune up your mood.

**Reduce your stress level**: Unwanted assignments and commitments give us stress and worries. So, prioritize them as early as you can. Get organised them also. It will save your time and give you more opportunities for mellow moments. If you are stress-free, you feel yourself strong, energetic and sexy.

**Get enough sleep**: Lack of sleep is extremely dangerous. It can wreak havoc on your entire body, system and make you feel more stressed and sickened. If you don't have enough sleep of minimum six hours, you might not be able to enjoy the sexual activity.

**Yoga or meditation**: Regular practice of yoga and meditation also reduce stress and tension. It relaxes both our body and mind. When you are free from tension, you will be getting more libido power.

**Laughter**: It's often said that laughter is an excellent stress reliever. It delivers great benefits to our body and soul. So, try to wind down with a funny TV show or an interesting fiction book which gives you hilarious laughs. Always share some jokes with some on love, it will sparkle your heart and prompt your desires.

**No detachment**: After the birth of a new baby, ladies are often preoccupied with its care and forget the spouse. They are fully connected to the newborn baby. Such detachment in spousal relationships is quite detrimental. I would suggest ladies to spare some time for their spouse for amorous conversations. Enjoy your adult life fully.

**Getting romantic with music** If you are cheerless for some trivial reason, don't get confused. Music, dance, aromatherapy or playing carom or ludo with your spouse can help you refresh your mood. It can help you in relaxing and give you a mood of getting romantic.

## Chapter Eighteen

## Tooth Tips for Pregnant Ladies

Most expected mothers only think about the deficiencies of essential iron and see the gynecologists to take their advice to fight off the iron deficiency but they forget that the care of teeth is also needed for them during pregnancy due to repeatedly vomiting and certain other health reasons

Have you ever thought about taking extra care of teeth during pregnancy? Most expected mothers only think about the deficiencies of essential iron and see the gynecologists to take their advice regarding it. They perhaps know, during pregnancy, more calcium is needed for child's bones?

And it is said that calcium is pulled out from teeth for this purpose. Although it is a myth yet there is no denying that the care of teeth is needed for the pregnant ladies due to a few certain reasons.

Actually, once calcium is deposited in the teeth that can never be pulled out at any circumstances but teeth need more care during pregnancy because ladies generally, during this period, become careless. Once the lady conceives, she begins to feel morning nausea or sickness, often several times a day.

Ladies generally feel exhausted and vomit repeatedly. They avoid doing extra work because ill health at time forces them to take it easy.

Sheer exhaustion also makes a woman casual regarding the cleanliness of the body parts. They more often than not find themselves in no mood to brush their teeth also. Moreover, repeated acidic vomiting tarnishes the enamel of the teeth. Vomiting causes the teeth an enormous damage similarly that happens to the floor marble exposed to the acid. What is more, for the development of embryo, most ladies are prone to eating repeatedly which in fact is not good for the health of their teeth.

If a pregnant woman eats frequently, she invites the chances of increasing cavities. It is a truth, the more the ladies eat, the more they invite cavities. If one eats more than five times a day, she will be prone to more dental cavities. Having good teeth plus maintaining good oral hygiene is good for the unborn child.

If you have cleaner teeth, you will have lesser disease producing bacteria in your mouth. If your teeth are bad, you may probably transmit disease producing bacteria to your child.

It is better for you to eat less sweetened things, foodstuff, drinks etc. during pregnancy. The ladies should take even more care of their teeth making some extra efforts and spending more time in the upkeep of their teeth because during this period, hormonal balance gets disturbed.

They should do regular brushing. Ladies experience "pregnancy gingivitis" when they are more prone to gum disease due to lack of tooth care. Bad gums sometimes become the cause of underweight child. Some women experience the growth on their gums also.

In medical terms, we call this growth "pregnancy tumor". Although, such kinds of tumors are regressed routinely after the delivery but if the ladies try to get it removed during pregnancy, it can occur again after the removal. The best way to erase the acid on your teeth is dry brushing. Pregnant ladies should brush their teeth without toothpaste for about five to ten minutes then spit out to remove the bacteria from their mouth and then brush their teeth with paste for cleansing the teeth. Expected mothers! I suggest you clean your teeth after each vomit and ensure that no germs are passed to the unborn child. Why don't you adopt good habit? Do you really want a sick child?

## Chapter Nineteen

### Care your heart in winter

The risk of having a heart attack in winter is more twice than the summer and moreover, the attacks in winter are more likely to be fatal. Do you know how to care your heart in winter?

In India, very few people know that in winter months, there is an increase of about twenty percent or more incidences of cardiac arrests than summer months. Reason is quite simple; we are not used to living in artificially regulated temperatures.

In peak winter season, temperature plummets even to below five degree Celsius and for those who are already suffering some heart diseases, the time is more risky than the commoners.  The more we prevent ourselves from being exposed to cold, the better it will be for the wellbeing of our hearts.

### Why the heart attacks are more in winter

In winter months, when a person gets exposed to cold wintry weather, his blood vessels narrow to the skin to retain heats to the body but for the patients of heart diseases who have arteries already filled with plague, the risk of heart attacks increases for those patients.

In such condition, not only the heart have to work harder but the blood supply to the heart also is reduced which becomes the reason of cardiac arrest. Moreover, in winter months, blood platelets appear to be more active and stickier and, therefore, more likely to clots. Even the level of cholesterol rises in the months of winters. These all are the prelude to heart attack. Now, it is only you who better know how you can protect your heart in winter. Doctor can only advise you.

## Be cautious if you have weak heart

Friends! If you are a heart patient, winter is really a bad time for you if you are casual and not careful. Several medical studies show that in winter, even the person with normal heart feels the increased level of stress.

If you have a weak heart, obviously; the danger for you may be more. A research report published in a journal by American Heart Association says that the rate of heart disease related deaths from December 25 to January 7 is higher.

These are the days of peak winter and in this season, people tend to eat and drink more. They gain more weight which triggers cardiac arrest.

## How to Reduce the Risk

I suggest if you are the patients of heart, you must take some common sense preventive measures to safeguard your hearts. People with a build up of fatty plaque are more prone to cardiac diseases. Smoking, hypertension, high cholesterol, diabetes and the lack of exercise are the prime reasons which trigger cardiovascular diseases. So, avoid such foods which allow your bodies to retain fats and cholesterol.

## Sunshine vitamin D

Remember, basking in the sun and drinking a plenty of milk can reduce the risk of cardiac arrest. Sun basking is the best source of vitamin D. Body makes vitamin D in sufficient amount when exposed to sunlight. It is the best source to protect the heart but our typical Indian diet doesn't provide enough vitamin D. For getting vitamin D, you can take orange juice, cereals and some particular types of foods which we routinely can't afford.

But people over sixty needs to take more vitamin D supplements because old people have a higher risk for vitamin D deficiencies. Aging itself makes it harder for the body to make Vitamin D and convert it to a useable form.

## Useful tips to stay away from heart diseases

1.	Always go for morning and evening walk. Always stay active to brave the cold weather but avoid very early morning and late evening walk. Let the sun rise. In evening walk, don't wait for the sun to set and protect you from chilly wind. Never expose to very cold temperature.

2.	Avoid fatty, fried and non vegetarian food. Never binge on nuts and dry fruits also.

3.	Moreover, avoid alcohol, smoking and caffeine. Maybe, they give you a sense of warmth for the time being but don't forget; they stimulate the heart and can cause high blood pressure.

4.	If you are preoccupied with your home duties and unable to go out for walk regularly, do active in your household chores like sweeping, cleaning, mopping and washing clothes without using the washing machine. Likewise, indoor activity like dancing and water aerobics can keep you fit and stay away from heart diseases.

5       At home, you can work out with hand weights or stretch bands to enhance your resistance power to fight against the diseases. Such exercises can be done while you are watching your favourite TV programmes or listening to the music.

6       You can join a health club or gym and use machines like treadmills, stair climber or exercise bikes to stay you fit and healthy.

7       If you feel any chest pain, immediately call on doctor. Don't postpone the treatment. Maybe, it is muscular pain but don't take it lightly.

8       If you have sedentary jobs for long hours, don't use the lift while you go for office or come back, walk on stairs the maximum you can do, it will be an extra activity even on your busy work schedule.

## Dress for cold months

1       Most ladies wear sleeveless clothes when they go out for attending a wedding ceremony in winter months; it is not an ideal fashion statement in such weather. For outdoor activities, wear clothes which are made of pure wool and polypropylene. They should be fit well so that keep you warm and dry.

2       Also, don't forget wear socks with waterproof shoes but remember they should fit in closely but not be too tight.

3       If there is foggy season or chilly winds are blowing, wear warm cap or muffler. You should also wear covering for your face such as a scarf.

If you are a patient of heart disease. Don't forget to cover your head and chest. A monkey cap may give you funny look but it is best cloth for the protection of both head and face.

## Chapter Twenty

### Laser Touch for Beauty

How much do you love pampering yourself? Have you heard about laser touch, a new trend in medical spa? The word laser is the latest buzz in beauty industry. This strong weapon that eradicates the skin scars of every sort- is a new journey of aesthetic technology in skin rejuvenation solutions

Pragmatically, it is one of the best and effective solutions for all beauty ailments, despite being the most expensive one. The most common use of laser is for hair removal, tattoo removal, birth marks removal, stretch marks removal, pigmentation removal, skin rejuvenation and tightening etc.

Sometimes, when blood vessels settle on the surface of the skin, dermatologists advise their patients or clients for its reduction through laser, to give a new look to the skin.

However, some people think that laser touch always has several side effects and it is a riskier and unsafe method, because it gives the patients painful or irritating sensation similar to the clunk of rubber band against the skin, or the sting of several piercing needles in the body, which stays forever. There is also a risk of some bacterial infections in the body, which invite other skin diseases at later stage.

### What the doctors opine

While talking to several doctors, I learnt if one seeks a licensed practitioner or a well-trained dermatologist, and approved laser is used in the right frequency, then there is no harm in going in for laser treatment. Laser hair removal, for people with darker skin, may be more difficult and more painful.

After treatment, the laser-touched area generally swells, turns slightly discoloured for one to five or six days, but there is rare chance of permanent discoloration or scarring. Tattoo removal is also a more painful exercise, but the results of laser treatment are always positive.

In hair removal laser treatment, low-energy beams are sent into the skin which is absorbed by darker pigmented areas. The laser energy after some time becomes heated and destroys the roots of the hair properly so that it doesn't grow again.

It is the slow process and is done carefully. People, who have lighter skin or darker hair or both, can enjoy the best and quick benefits of this treatment. One must understand that laser treatments can be made painless. With absolute care, blistering can, no doubt, be avoided.

If one experiences swelling and redness, he should not be afraid. Such short-term side effects are because of laser's heat, nothing else. Generally, 48 hours before starting a full treatment, practitioners conduct a test on a small area of skin, to watch its effects on the skin. Moreover, lasers too are equipped with skin cooling devices. Doctors generally suggest the patients to use a cool-pack on the laser inflicted area, to reduce pain after treatment, but despite that, if the patient thinks or the surgeon notices that the skin is over sensitive, he should apply anesthetic cream before the treatment or discuss everything with the doctors.

## No cheaper salon package

Some people opt for cheaper salon packages. They generally stay away from visiting an experienced, reputed and certified dermatologist, because hair reduction takes much time, almost 10-12 sittings, and each sitting is very expensive. They don't want to pay more, so they put their life into peril.

Those, who are already affected with herpes, should tell the doctors prior to the treatment. Antiviral medication should also be provided to such patients, to avoid abnormal scarring; otherwise, continuing negative side effects of laser hair removal are very rare.

Before going in for laser touch, you must keep two things in your mind. First, let the doctors or healthcare provider know everything abut your specific circumstances; second, always avoid going in for cheaper treatment because it can give more loss than benefit.

If one fails to hire a qualified person and a sterilized system, there are strong chances of getting bacterial infections.

## It all depends on skin types

Most cosmetic surgery consultants opine that, for Indian skins, they have to work carefully, despite knowing that there is a low or no risk in laser peels. In laser peel, the upper layer of the skin is removed. For a peel, the top layer of the skin is removed by laser. It gives flash burn to the skin.

There are type-four and type-five skin types. After laser peel is done on Indian skin, the recovery time is always high. Indians have mostly dark skin tone and the patients of such sort of skin take much longer time to recover. So, it should be done judiciously otherwise there are strong chances of post inflammatory hyper pigmentation.

## Keep off bleaching and facial

Generally, beauty conscious ladies frequently visit beauty parlors for facial, bleaching etc. They should keep away from such beauty treatments for at least five-six weeks, after the laser skin treatment done. It is much risky and such practice should be shunned.

Laser treatment is done to rejuvenate the skin, so; the skin takes some time to recover itself. After the treatment, one has to use mild cleansers and antiseptics. Also, one should never use medicated soaps or creams, after the laser treatment, for some time.

## Discuss every issue with dermatologists

Every client should understand the procedure and discuss every issue regarding laser touch, before going in for the treatment. He should also discuss the results he desires and what his/her expectations are from the treatment.

Although, this procedure has no connection with cancer, as it is preached by some misinformed people, and there is no fear of penetration in the body tissues; yet everyone should ensure full knowledge about the procedure, precautions and post treatment care etc.

Moreover, the wisdom and skill of the person who administers the treatment matters a lot. On the basis of my conversation with several doctors, I can conclude that laser touch procedure entails a series of non-invasive treatments at particular body points plus direct treatment of unwanted wrinkles.

## Who should not go for laser touch?

- ✓ Pregnant Women should never seek laser procedure. It can damage foetus.
- ✓ Those who have skin tan should get rid of the tan before going for laser treatment, for getting quick results.
- ✓ The women who use alcohol frequently should take precaution before opting for laser touch.
- ✓ Antiviral medicine should also be taken before the treatment.
- ✓ Clients taking Tetracycline, Retin and photosynthesizing medication should not go for laser treatment. First, they should stop medicine for several weeks prior to the laser touch treatment, then consult the doctor.
- ✓ The patients of diabetes should avoid laser treatment, or they must consult the specialists prior to the treatment.
- ✓ During fever or in high/low blood pressure, laser treatment is risky.

✓ Thorough body's check up is necessary before the treatment.

## General side effects of laser touch

Generally, laser treatment is considered to be safe and risk free; and its side effects are short-lived, provided the medico giving the treatment is quite experienced and well trained. But, the clients should also be aware of the side effects.

If one takes some precautions, he/she need not to be worried about the side effects. In 2005, a female patient from North Carolina had died during treatment because of the application of some extra quantity of anesthetic cream on the preferred area before starting the process.

So, don't do such things before consulting the doctors. Always remember the following points.

✓ Don't ever consume some extra doze of medicine without the prescription of senior specialists.

✓ This method of cure can develop blisters on the upper part of the lips. In medical terminology, it is known as FEVER BLISTER. Do be afraid of it.

✓ After the treatment, swelling and mild redness surfaces, despite the proper manner of treatment by experts. Always remember, it is a natural process.

✓ One can experience skin irritations and feelings of pain.

✓ After the treatment, one experiences the lightening or darkening of his/her skin. It is only for the time being.

✓ Dark-skin people are likely to get many blisters after treatment and they might take a long period to fade away.

## Laser treatment for wrinkles

The clinical protocol for laser touch is designed with different programmes viz. skin rejuvenation, scar tissue; improve skin moisture levels; acne and facial wrinkles etc. This treatment improves the efficiency of the body, anti-aging system and the organ system. All it is achieved through an absolutely natural mechanism.

Daniel Ward and Shan Baker; noted dermatologists of USA had once said that the treatment of facial wrinkles with carbon dioxide laser is a well established and successful way of eliminating wrinkles. They had also accepted that there are side effects such as darkening and lightening of the skin, with this treatment, but one should not worry, as, after some time, the skin automatically restores its previous place.

Here, it's important to mention that in laser treatment, carbon dioxide is used and laser vaporizes water molecules inside and outside the cells. The process causes thermal damage on the surrounding tissues. In this process, the skin produces more protein collagen, which fills the wrinkles. In this treatment, there are chances of eruption of herpes simplex virus, which later becomes the reason of skin blistering, sores etc.

## Laser treatment for whitening teeth

These days, laser dentistry has become popular for various purposes such as cavity removal, gum reshaping, teeth whitening etc. It is helpful in several other aspects of dental health practice also. Moreover, it gives less pain and minimizes recovery time also.

The most advanced method, at present, is the adoption of laser teeth-whitening procedure. It is undoubtedly one of the best dental solutions, with which, one can rejuvenate the colour of his/her teeth. It's no doubt, at present; it's the safest as well as the fastest way to get the teeth whitened. In this treatment, a unique laser whitening gel is administered to a person's teeth, followed by high intensity laser to penetrate the whitening materials into the teeth.

Before the treatment, you must have to tell the dentist your complete previous history and talk to him about your expectations of results. No doubt, whitening of teeth is a straightforward procedure, but you must make sure that the dentist who is doing the procedure is qualified and has appropriate knowledge of advanced techniques.

## Laser treatment for carpal tunnel syndrome

Laser treatment for carpal tunnel syndrome is a unique technique involving the use of some lights to stimulate the tissues, blood flow and the release of natural chemicals to cure the ailment. For this treatment, a qualified and expert doctor is required. Moreover, this treatment is much expensive, so you should go for this surgery, only if the doctors declare that the other non-invasive treatments have remained unsuccessful.

One should wear eye protection goggles during laser therapy session as the laser is focused on the wrist, which is close by the eyes. Generally, specialists tell the patients how to protect their eyes. Second, one should try to hold his/her hands as still as possible, so as the light which penetrate through two inches of the body, could always remain focused. Some patients want quick result but it is not possible in the carpal tunnel syndrome. The treatment takes some weeks and several sittings.

**Laser touch for acne removal**

Laser touch for acne removal is a popular method of getting rid of acne or unwanted angry pimples. It is a very welcome development. In the old method of acne treatment, acnes leave unsightly and even disfiguring scars behind, but with laser touch, the science of acne scar removal has evolved significantly.

In old time, dermabrasion was a preferred method of removing acnes, in which scarred uppermost layer of the skin was removed. In this method, doctors administer anesthesia first. After dermabrasion, the skin looks raw and unsightly. This procedure is quite painful and very irritating. In the past, many doctors used chemical peels to remove scars. The use of chemicals causes the skin to blister and finally peel off; so, this procedure is also quite drastic and much agonizing.

With these laser procedures, the doctor retains total control over the procedure and no blood loss takes place. With the use of no-ablative laser, the affected surface of the skin is not burnt off; rather, surgeon burns off the scarred skin cells. After that, fresh skin cells replace burnt cells. Surgeons who perform laser-based acne scar removal operation should be highly qualified and must have considerable artistic ability.

## Chapter Twenty One

### Sleep Right

*Sometimes, when you wake up morning, your neck feels stiff or you experience a severe pain in your back and experience a general lethargic feeling. If you visit the doctor, he may prescribe you some anti-inflammatory pain killer medicine. Maybe, you will be advised hot water therapy. However, these are not permanent solutions of your body discomfort. Then, where is the problem? Have you ever thought of your method of sleeping? If not, improve your method and recover your health. I'm sure; sleeping right is the only way that may help you from these ailments.*

First thing, think of the pillow you use, while you sleep. Is it right? Does it provide adequate support for your neck? In most cases, pillows are the chief cause of causing a pain in the neck. Doctors say that a pillow which is neither soft nor hard is always the ideal choice. The pillow must be placed under the upper shoulder, extend till the head and shoulder support the interior curve of the neck, crushing to fit inside neck curvature.

If the pillow is very soft it might not support the head, while a hard pillow also won't be able to support the neck at the right angle. The right choice would be to buy carefully contoured pillows.

Remember, when you lay on your back you can place soft pillow beneath your knees for your comfort. Some people lay on their stomach. For them, placing a pillow beneath chest may be comfortable. The size of the pillows should be equivalent to the width and height of the body configuration.

## Keep your "back" in original shape

An Irish Proverb goes, "A good laugh and a long nap are the best cures in the doctor's book. If your "back" doesn't get proper comfort from the mattress you choose, you can't enjoy your morning. "Back" is most important part of the body which needs total relaxation and the mattress you choose has to help you achieve this.

Our back has also a curve which needs to be supported. The right mattress is important. It must adapt to one's body shape when he/she lies on it. Moreover, it must be made of coir fibre. Remember when you wake up in the morning; your back must be in its original shape. You must change the mattress every three four years because the coir fibre loses its flexibility after three four years.

## Some Essentials

For a good night sleep and to wake up to a healthy morning.

- ✓ Eat light food; avoid excessive alcohol.

- ✓ Exercise regularly, as it encouraged deeper sleep and reduces stress hormones.

- ✓ Don't sleep where there is noise and bright lights, as it will disturb your sleep frequently. Use heavy curtains to reduce light and earplugs to minimize noise.

- ✓ Always keep your bedroom ventilated and at a comfortable temperature.

- ✓ Don't take long nap in the afternoons if you want to sleep early at night.

- ✓ Go to bed and get up in the morning at fixed time.

- ✓ Before going to bed, relax your body, wash your face; brush your teeth. This will mentally prepare you for going to bed.

- ✓ Keep your mind off worries at the time of sleep and listen to soft music.

- ✓ Don't smoke; consume alcohol, at least four hours before bedtime.

- ✓ Never discuss emotional issues, while in bed.

- ✓ Avoid watching TV or work on laptop, while you in your bed. Remember, the bed is only for sleeping.

- ✓ If you are on the bed for 20-30 minutes and still awake, don't try to sleep forcibly. Get up and start to work or read a book until you feel a bit drowsy. Some people encourage the myth of the right/wrong sleep posture. Actually, when one goes to sleep, he doesn't know what the right posture is. Every posture is right and fine if it gives you complete relaxation.

## Chapter Twenty Two

## Pills without Prescription

*Most ladies consider 'appointment-with-the doctor' as a futile exercise. "What is the need to seek doctor's prescription and waste time" Even when the pills are available everywhere and chemists can tell you how and when you should have to take them. Do you know the contraceptive pills- without the prescription are more dangerous than good?*

Thanks to the advertisements in print media and TV channels, we generally notice ladies visiting chemist shops to buy pills which are without any prescription from gynecologist. Such pills are easily available at every medical store. If you are one of them, you can spoil your health.

## Every pill is not for every woman

Here, it is agonizing to mention, as per medical report almost 70 percent ladies skip the appointment with the gynecologist and get any pill that the drugstores provide them. Do you know 'over-the-drugstores contraceptive pills' could be more dangerous? Such practice may give the ladies a series of horrible ailments.

Every lady owns a different body type, so the pill available at drugstore may not suit everyone, thus doctor's advice is must. Pills in the market contain different levels of hormones. Some have the combination of estrogen and progestin, while others contain only progestin. Due to different hormones structure, it is difficult for everyone to opt for the right medicine without doctor's advice. Remember, every pill is not for every lady.

## Before The Prescription

Before we prescribe a pill, we take different tests from hormonal to blood pressure. Eating and smoking habits and exercise routine of the patient is also enquired. We inquire about patients' family history.

It helps us to decide on which pill is better for the particular lady. One type of pill may help woman in improving her skin but the other type may ruin the skin with rashes and acnes.

I must suggest ladies to consult their doctors at least for first three months and check their weight and blood pressure as well to keep their health, for all time, in good condition.

We generally hear some women complaint of irregular periods, high blood pressure, weight gain, depression, headache and stomach cramps etc. I think it is due to wrong medication apart from lack of care of the body.

Some ladies have more male hormones; therefore, they should consume pills, which contain only estrogen. For such ladies, pills containing progestin and estrogen can worsen their hormonal balance.

## Regular schedule is must

For the effectiveness of the pills, regularity is must. You must take the pill exactly as advised by your physician. One should take the pill at the same time everyday without gap. Fix a time for it. (Fix an alarm/ reminder)

The best time for taking the medicine is one or two hours after the meals. In the first few weeks, ladies might experience nausea but it goes away with the time.

If you have some other ailments such as diarrhea, fever or vomiting during the menstrual cycle and you are taking the medicine for those ailments also, then the effectiveness of the pills is most likely reduced, so it is better to use some other contraceptives such as condoms for protection in that period.

Generally, the combination of progestin and estrogen is 99 percent effective but in some ladies, we observe the bodies of some patients don't react well to the estrogen in the combined pill, so we have to give them the only progestin pills for better results.

## Chapter Twenty Three

## Back Pain after Work

As women and men cross their thirties, they begin to feel something convulsing inside the lower portion of their chest. The main reason of the back pain is pressure on the roots of the nerves. Prolonged sitting or fall on hips can lead to muscle spasm exerting pressure on sciatic nerve.

Due to pressure, numbness in the back occurs and causes pain. After work for long hours, back pain is commonplace phenomenon. Do you know how you can overcome it?

**Tips to remove back pain after work -**

**"Back Pain" After Work**

Most women and men often complain of a back pain after doing some work. There are several reasons for it, but it starts due to fatigue or minor pain in your legs. Sometimes legs ache is experienced without any injury, which later causes pain in the back. Due to tiredness, sometimes pain radiates from leg to lower back or hips etc. It may prolong to several months.

It may be either due to nerve problem or vascular affliction. It often happens when sciatic nerve is pressed. "Sciatica (a term for pain radiation) is not a disorder but a symptom of several problems involving the nerves.

Due to hectic lifestyle and imbalanced diet, one can become the patient of back pain even in young age but after thirty, it is common to both men and women if they have sedentary habits. Just after crossing the thirty, one may begin to feel something convulsing inside the lower portion of their chest.

The main reason of the back pain is pressure on the roots of the nerves. Prolonged sitting or fall on hips can lead to muscle spasm exerting pressure on sciatic nerve. Due to pressure, numbness in the back occurs and causes pain.

## How to reduce back pain

1. Take pain killer to reduce pain and inflammation but be careful while taking it. Take the very pain killer which acclimatizes your body. Don't take any pain killer without consulting the doctor.
2. Relaxation for 24 hours to 48 hours may relieve severe back pain.
3. Don't rest for more than two three days. Inactivity may cause muscle weakness.
4. Don't lift heavy objects while doing daily domestic chores.
5. Don't do activities like forward bending or backward bending. It may intensify your pain.
6. Use hot packs if doctor advises you.
7. Do light exercise to promote your body releasing endorphins which stops pain signals from reaching the brain.
8. When the pain decreases after medicines, start with some exercises, which will improve the posture and flexibility strengthening your muscles, after consulting experts.
9. Walking regularly and running on a stationary bicycle is essential. These activities will help you stay active.

## Care at home

1. Lie on your back with pillow under the knees or hips.
2. Sleep on the side with bent knees or pillow between your knees; sleep on a firm mattress or on a wooden cot.
3. Place a rolled towed behind the back when sitting on chair, for added comfort.
4. Bend your knees when lifting any object from the ground.
5. Try to keep your back straight, holding the object close to the body.
6. You should not try to lift any object beyond the capacity. They should take firm mattress or sleep on wooden cot.

## Remember

When the pain becomes intolerable, don't do home made medications. Contact the doctor immediately and ask for essential epidural steroid injection.

It is the only way to reduce inflammation and severe pain. For long time relief in life, don't forget three injections every year

## Chapter Twenty Four

### Sugar Free Diet

*After forty, most of us begin to worry about sugar point in our bodies. Due to our hectic lifestyle and redundant food and drink habits, we often gain some extra weight. We then begin to think that sugar free diet is the only solution to get rid of our extra pounds.*

*Medicos term the sugar free diet as diabetic diet. There is no denying that diabetic patients have to resort to sugar free diet. No doubt, sugar free diet helps us in stabilizing our blood sugar levels, weight control, dental problem and several other diabetic related ailments including vision disorder but remember that sugar is also the need of the body.*

Here, we should well understand that sugar free diet implies getting rid of dreadful forms of sugar which are found in delicious candies, sweetmeat, cakes, beverages and more cups of tea/coffee which have high sugar contents but empty calories.

The more use of toffees, sweets and candies often leads to dental problem viz. tooth decay and gum diseases.

In the name of sugar free diet, we sometimes begin to avoid good sugars which are naturally found in fruits and honey and weaken our bodies by not providing the calories to our bodies which are essentially needed.

If you are one of such persons, don't forget the need of sugar for your body and understand my focus- 'all about is not good for sugar free diet'.

## Facts about sugar free cookies

We daily see several people who are dreaming to shed extra pounds, buying packs of sugar free cookies or blobs of fat free butter in the market.

Several reports and studies show that these food packs are not only hopeless in helping lose weight but they also lead to deficiencies in our body.

These free sugar foods are generally low calories and may be health hazard. I don't say unpleasant words for these products but I must suggest you, it would be better if you consult the doctor before buying such products.

## Disadvantages of SFD

SFD- sugar free diet contains sucralose. If one takes overdose of sucralose he/she has to experience headaches and dizziness. There are strong chances of depression and anxiety if one often consumes sugar free foods.

Generally, people buy fat free food to shed their pounds but fat is a necessary nutrient they forget while doing so. Eating fat free food means missing important nutrients which your body necessarily requires.

Don't ever make it a big part of your diet otherwise you definitely will end up with a score of deficiencies.

## Avoid excessive use of fat free food

We all know that fat gives the food a good taste. When the fat is taken out from the food, it becomes tasteless; then to provide it the taste, some chemicals such as monosodium glutamate and sugar are added to it. The excessive use of such foods is harmful. It results in insulin resistance and even diabetes.

Moreover, such fat-free foods don't give satisfaction. People tend to eat such food more and more to delight their appetite. So, it becomes worse than eating "full of fat" food. So, avoid it as maximum as you can.

Natural sources of sugar are ideal

If  you want to keep away from sugar,  you ought to choose the natural sources of it such as honey, fruits and maple syrups etc. Body requires requisite calories, so; to get the necessary calories, go for real foods- full of natural proteins and fats which essentially will be helpful in satisfying you.

Maintaining good health is the basic need of the body and for this one has to satisfy the basic nutritional needs of the body with balanced diet so as the body could function efficiently.

If one generally chooses milk, yoghurt, cheese, poultry, meats, fish and fruits and every kind of veggies, he/she needs not to be worried over their sugar level in the body. You might be surprised to find out that most people do not lose weight with sugar-free diets foods. They may gain weight instead.

## Sugar: from health view point

From a health viewpoint, sugar is valueless as it contains no nutrition. If one doesn't take sugar to make his/her taste different, there might be the slightest harm to the body. People see it as a danger to blood glucose levels but, in actuality, most high sugar foods don't raise blood glucose levels as compared to bread like starchy foods.

## Importance of sugar

Sugar has, no doubt, bad reputation if one intends to lose weight. But one should never overreact and stop eating sugar altogether. We should assess how important sugar is for our health and in our routine diet. We always should take it at reasonable level. Sugar is best and concentrated source of energy.

Medical study says that the energy value of sugar is quite high. One gram sugar gives 4 calories minimum. If you are looking for short term energy boost, rational use of sugar is ideal. Moreover, sugar floods us with pleasure.

It stimulates the release of the neurotransmitter serotonin and probably other mood-elevating substances also. As per reports from different quarters, brain response in eating sugar is as quick as falling in love.

Moreover, the special taste of sweet food generates enzymes which provides extra boost to our brain.

## Prevalent in every food

Actually, absolute sugar free diet is a misnomer term. Weight loss success with such diets is rare. You may think you are taking sugar free diet.

But, actually what we take in our daily routine, every food except for water and meat contains some amount of sugar. Do you live only on water and meat? Perhaps not. Even soda which is used in our food items also contains some sugar.

Sugar free puddings which are sold in markets contain about six grams of sugar plus at least 80-90 calories. Wine and alcohol are also sugar. Having a glass of wine is equal to a daily-served sweet dish altogether.

## Sugar level in sugar free diets

On the labels of almost all sugar free diets, we generally read some words- such as glucose, corn syrup, dextrose, lactose, fructose, sucrose, maltose and honey etc. All these words indicate that there is some form of sugar in all these products. Moreover, sugar is a kind of carbohydrate and they (carbohydrates) are often found in every type of food which comes from plants either they are vegetables, grains, fruits or legumes.

Additionally, milk products such as yoghurt and milk itself too have carbohydrates. Carbohydrates are our need to boost our energy level that one should often take in healthy carbohydrates food. If one chooses healthy foods he/she needs not to resort to sugar free diets.

## In the favour of polyols

Several doctors talk in favour of such foods which contain "polyols". Polyols is another name of sugar alcohols but they are neither sugars nor alcohols. They are a group of low digestible carbohydrates which taste like sugar. No doubt, such foods are good but if you indulge in over-consumption of polyols-containing foods, there are strong chances of gastrointestinal disorders and laxative effects.

## Advantages of polyols

Here, let me tell you the advantages of polyols

1 Polyols is a sweetened- sugar free food

2 It is a low calorie food

3 It serves a useful substitute of sugar

4 Polyols prevent tooth decay

5 Polyols are also used in toothpastes and mouthwashes

6 These are also used in cough syrups and throat lozenges

7 Polyols don't cause abrupt increase in blood sugar levels

8 Polyols help people in achieving body weight loss

## Sugar's side effect

In our routine life, we often take on much sugar for which our bodies are not ready to accept. It is a proven truth that sugar is very hard to digest. For its digestion, our bodies have to work harder. Overeating of sugar triggers several ailments in our bodies such as constant headache, tooth decay, indigestion; early menopause, hormonal imbalance, migraines, insomnia, depression, aggression, irritability etc.

## In a Nutshell

Artificial packed sweeteners are more chemicals less food! They have no calories because they don't nourish our body in anyway — they're indeed toxins our body gathers. If one doesn't live without these packaged diets, use it but you should be careful and give your body some extra supports elsewhere.

## Chapter Twenty Five

## Overcome Your Depression

*Down to several constant failures in life, some times, we feel that we are just living a worthless and hollow life. Neither we eat properly nor sleep soundly and always think negatively. Even sometimes, we misconstrue that Almighty God is our foe.*

*If this situation endlessly continues more than two week and hinders normal activities of your routine life, you must understand that you immediately need to contact the doctor and explain him your condition. You may be suffering from the silent killer known as depression*

Psychiatrists opine that there are some kinds of feelings that haunt every one at some point in time. To overcome the feelings, one needs to first understand its causes.

Needless to say that some negative feelings of unhappiness, frustration and worry are common to all people and they don't affect significantly our abilities to perform routine duties. Such feelings rather help us to understand our weak points. Grief and miseries help us to face the adversity of our life in a better way. Don't misinterpret such feelings as depression.

### What is depression?

Don't be scared everybody has to experience failures in life. Generally, people overcome their failures by the time. Time itself is a great healer. In failure situations, sleeplessness and lack of appetite are common symptoms.

But if your grief, instead of decreasing by the time, becomes more intense and lasts more than two three weeks, you should understand that you have reached at the depressed state of mind. In such situations, you need the help of psychiatrist.

Don't forget that the major characteristics of depression are not only the presence of negative feelings but the long intensity and long duration also.

**How to ascertain you are depressed**

1.  When you feel yourself totally weak without any inclination to do anything.
2.  When you have the feeling of fear from your neighbours or friends.
3.  When you retain the feeling that you will never cure in your life.
4.  When you feel that you are unable to fight against your disease with courage and willpower.
5.  When you only see the bad side of things and feel that something ghastly is going to be happened with you and such feelings haunt you again and again.
6.  When you give more attention to your errors focusing your attention primarily on the number of errors you have made.
7.  When you feel the continuous feelings of grief, stress, anxiety, frustration and indecision.
8.  When you have the feelings of more or less appetite for food and loss of your energy and the feeling of exhaustion.
9.  When you have the feeling of being guilty.
10. When you are resorted to the feeling of isolation
11. When you lose the interest or pleasure in all activities even in sex and lovemaking.

12      When you resort to the pessimistic feelings of death and suicide

13      When you have the feeling of headache or pain in your shoulder or any part of the body

## Doctor's opinion

I have consulted several doctors about depression and came to know that there are several different manifestations of depression which cause to destroy the conscience of victims. The earlier you thwart the depression, the better it would be for you.

Depression needs to be combated with caution before it shows the fury of its destructive actions. Depressed persons need the love, care and most importantly the supports of friends and family so; the family should always come forward to understand the feelings of the depressed person.

Certainly, with the help and guidance of a specialist, depression can be tackled. If the patient change the way of his/her thinking, he/she can protect him/herself from depression and doctors do such counseling apart from medication.

It is not a short term treatment. The experts in cognitive behavioral therapy are able to do such treatments.

### Treatment @ Home

1      Wake up in the morning when you are full of energy and go for morning walk immediately.

2      Stop feeling sad and think positively.

3      Stop crying over trivial issues.

4       Try to be free from drugs because its constant use affects the body very much

5       Improve your confidence. It is the natural way to overcome depression

6       Always hope for better life in future. If you think better, the things will improve automatically. If you think negatively, the things will worsen.

7       Be strong and courageous against despair. It is the better way to fight the depression

8       Change your attitude. The world will follow you and you will be happy with the world.

9       Tell yourself you are better and try to believe that, and then you will see you are really in a better position.

## Chapter Twenty Six

## Keep Yourself Fit in Summer Season

Everyone wants to keep fit and healthy for all time. But, during summer months, we generally find ourselves in tight spot. Hot days spell trouble for us. In this season, we often think and plan to stay fit but didn't know how.

My suggestion for this 'season fitness' is: Always try to get protected from scorching, sweltering sun. Always take energy foods and drink plenty of water. Exercise wisely and rationally

## Start your day with water

In hot days, our body sweats more and becomes dehydrated quicker than any other season. To avoid dehydration, drink water plentifully. It will reload your lost fluids. Medical study says that drinking sufficient plain water in the morning, just after coming out of the bed is a good habit which will help you eradicating several ailments. Not only morning, drink water continuously throughout the day for the freshness of your skin.

It is even more important if you go for morning exercise in summer season. You can take sports drinks also. They will bring back the electrolytes that you have lost by sweating. While traveling, carry water bottle also. Eat fresh fruits and vegetables which are rich in vitamins and dietary fibre as well as good sources of water.

## Eat carefully

In winter season, you can eat whatever you fancy. But in summer season, eat very carefully, in a controlled and focused manner. In summer season, it is much better if you take smaller meals- five to six times throughout the day instead of two-three heavy meals.

Take the breakfast at 8 am, lunch at 1 pm and dinner at 7 pm. Meanwhile, you can take meager snacks at 11 am, 3 pm and 9 pm to give constant energy to your body.

This way, your body will be better able to use the food you have eaten time to time. It will help you in raising metabolism.

## Morning walk is essential

Exercise, either you do in the morning or in the evening, is good for the body and fitness but morning walk or exercise is much better for health. You must do some exercise right after you get out of the bed. If you have a stationary bicycle at home, don't forget running paddles on it both in the morning and in the evening.

Some people, due to scorching heat, abandon their fitness routine. You don't do so. If you are upset due to any reason, try to engage in some funny activities which could burn your calories giving you the overall fitness benefits.

Remember, the cycling is funny and low impact workout. It is a wonderful outdoor activity as well as exercise for beginners. You need not ride on bike to do errands if you want to see yourself fit and healthy.

## Swimming for cool-cool

In summer season, swimming is the best option to burn calories. It is both a fun and a workout. It helps us in building upper and lower body strength.

Believe, in just a set of 30 minutes swimming, you can burn about 250 calories. Moreover, water relaxes the body. It is even better workout than exercise on ground.

## Take protein, drop carbohydrates

What you eat is equally important for the fitness of your body. Take protein in maximum amount in summer season; avoid carbohydrates if possible but don't forget that both protein and carbohydrates are essential energy foods for the body.

If you are worried about your weight gain, then discard fatty food completely. Fish, meats, eggs, beans, dairy products, soya and nuts are the best sources of protein but they are digested slowly so take such foods in a limited quantity.

## Protection from blistering sun

Protection from sweltering sun is also essential in summer months. It is a real threat for the body. Never do exercise in the sun. If you go outside between 10 am to 3 pm, you must wear sunglasses.  Also, wear sun protective clothes to protect your body.

## Chapter Twenty Seven

### Your Child's Teeth

Parents generally think that the baby teeth are temporary and are going to fall out after a period so they should not worry about the teeth of their children. Actually, it is misnomer term.

Dentists opine that these teeth play an important role in child's health and development because they enable the kids to chew the food properly and also help them to pronounce the all new words at the time of learning at school.

Moreover, early decay of kids' teeth can lead to permanent teeth growing in the cooked shape which distorts the attractive smile of the kids. Thus, take care for baby teeth since its beginning is essential

Parents are generally worried about the protection of their kids' teeth. As the children grow, they begin taking solid foods regularly. Parents delight seeing their kids eating.

No doubt, eating by children is a good habit but I don't favour repeated eating by children. Children generally consume more unwanted junk and sweetened food and invite dental problem.

A very few parents know that the problem of early childhood dental cavies arises just after the teeth make their appearance in child's mouth. Parents generally think that the baby teeth are temporary and are going to fall out after a period then why they worry about?

Actually, it is not the real picture. Dentists say that these teeth play an important role in child's health and development because they enable the kids to chew the food properly and also help them to pronounce the all new words at the time of learning at school. Moreover, early decay of kids' teeth can lead to permanent teeth growing in the cooked shape which distorts the attractive smile of the kids.

I suggest the parents they should take care of their child's teeth at the initial stage since the appearance of the first tooth in child's mouth to make the child's smile attractive and charming.

## Before the appearance of the first tooth

Generally, the first tooth of a new born baby comes at about six month of age. At the time of baby's birth, the oral cavity has only gum pad.

Most parents don't care about the gum pad as they think that the baby takes only liquids, so there is no chance of decay in the mouth. My suggestion is: parents should clean the gum pad from time to time by a wet piece of soft cloth.

As soon as any tooth appears in the mouth, parents should wipe it clean carefully. Piece of damp cotton can also be used. When five-six teeth appear, parents should assist their kids to brush the teeth regularly until they learn to use the brush on their own effectively.

## Don't share the spoon with the baby

Most parents share utensils with their children while feeding them. There are several mothers who clean the spoon of the baby with their tongue to taste everything before giving it to them. This is the best way to make it easy for the bacteria to enter the child's mouth. If you are caring mother and love your child, stop transmitting infection to your child this way. Don't forget kissing the child onto the lips also transmits infection.

## Check the thumb sucking habit

Thumb sucking is common practice among tots. Till the age of three or four, it is fine, but some children don't stop sucking their thumbs after that age and parents don't care about the bad habit of their children. If any child of more than four year sucks thumb discourage him. Thumb sucking habit can lead the mouth deformation and tooth alignment.

## Excessive feed and sugar causes dental caries

Most children love to eat sugary items. It also causes cavities. Don't allow your kids to eat sugary items more than five times a day. The frequency of intake of sugar stuff matters more than the amount of sugar consumed.

Epidemiologic studies show that the intake of meals or sugary items more than five times a day also leads to an increase in the number of cavities. When the child begins to weep most mothers thrust their breasts into the mouth of the child without knowing the actual reason of the weeping.

Such practice also leads to childhood dental cavities. Breast feeding should also be given at proper hours not only for the dental health of the baby but for the overall health of the child.

## When baby is less than two years

✓ Never lay your baby on bed with a bottle in his mouth. It can deform the teeth shape. Help him/her while he/she takes feed.
✓ Make sure the bottle is clean and dry.
✓ Don't dip the pacifier in honey to delight the baby when he/she is weeping. Children like sweet taste but its excessive use may cause tooth decay. Germs in honey can also make the child sick.
✓ Clean the nipples of bottle every time by washing with soap, rinsing carefully with clean water.

## Remember

✓ Inculcate the habit of brushing in your child by brushing your teeth before them twice a day.
✓ Teach them the proper way of brushing.
✓ Don't let your child swallow tooth paste. You dispense the toothpaste and also supervise brushing until the child is seven eight years old.
✓ Teach your child not to take sugary items frequently because tooth decay is caused by bacteria in the mouth interacting with sugar.
✓ Use fluoridated toothpaste immediately after the child learns to spit toothpaste out.

## Chapter Twenty Eight

### Good Eating Habits of Your Kids!

Most mummies and grannies often complain about the insufficient eating of their kids. They force them to eat more and more, not considering what they are gobbling them is the right kind of food stuff.

You also may be one of the parents who believe in the quantity of the foods stuffs rather than quality. Children need optimal nutrition to develop good health and sound mind. So, quality of the food matters much

Think, are you certainly providing proper nutrients to your toddlers through balanced diets? Some young children delight their parents by picking enough food despite that they are always in poor health. Pediatricians say that kids are better than adults in examining their hunger and fullness feelings.

If the parents supply them balanced diets, they rarely will tend to overeat. As responsible parents, you keep in mind the following points and eating habits of your kids to see them everlastingly in good health.

### Don't worry over the frequency of child's meals

Eat repeatedly is no doubt a bad habit. I don't favour it but for children it is okay because children are always engaged in physical activities. Generally, kids eat something every two hours.

Being a responsible parent, it is your responsibility to check the growth rate of your child from time to time. If it is not encouraging, meet the pediatrician quickly. If your kid is normally growing and getting enough calories, you need not to worry about him.

But, most kids avoid taking meal at usual meal times. Encourage them to take meal at proper time. Don't foster bad habits in your children if you want to see their proper development and physical growth. Ensure to provide your kid at least 300 calories to meet the need of their bodies and brains.

## Give your child enough time to eat

Generally, children require more time to eat their foods than their elders. Don't compare your quickness with them. Give them enough time to eat their diets. Let them chew the food properly and digest it.

Remember, little stomachs have little mouths. They can ape the eating style of their parents but don't force them to build their habit of eating fast. Moreover, don't let them eat in front of the TV or computer.

This way, they could not have learnt the good habit of eating in the right way and undergo indigestive ailments. Teach them the eating etiquettes and let them enjoy their foods with their own pace.

## Let the kids to taste new foods

For the good health of kids, motivate them to taste new nutritious foods. Children often resist tasting new foods. You can offer such foods early in the meal when they are quite hungry.

If the kids are not interested to take the new stuffs at the initial stage, don't force them to devour but you can try to give the new food together with his old favourite stuff.

Your child may wish noodles for breakfast, noodles for lunch and noodles for dinner. If you stop him taking such food, maybe, he would eat nothing.

Children like varieties. Serve them all types- milk, cheese, cereals, breads, green vegetables, fruits, meats etc. with noodles- the food of his choice but don't provide him all foods in one meal.

## Table manners are essential

Teach your kids' table manners as early as possible. Usually, kids are messy eaters. They spill more than they eat. Table manners and proper use of forks and spoons will help them to eat neatly.

Avoid using expensive utensils if you are with the children at dinning table. Use tiny size utensils to attract them towards foods. Make the area of the table quite safe where your kids sit for eating.

## Always keep these points in mind

- ✓ Due to slow growth or sickness, maybe your child doesn't feel hungry. Don't compel him/her to eat if he/she is not hungry.
- ✓ Don't let your child munch snack in big amounts as he/she won't feel hungry when the mealtime comes.
- ✓ Children are wondrous imitators. What you desire to get them eaten, eat you first.
- ✓ Don't give your child too much liquid- like juice or milk during the meal. It may fill his/her stomach leaving no space for food.
- ✓ Eat together with the child. Don't let him/her to eat alone. Mealtime should be a pleasant experience. You can have a pleasant conversation with him/her. It will create a feeling of warmth, love and security for the children.
- ✓ Call your child on table when meal is ready otherwise he/she will entertain himself/herself by playing and doesn't eat with concentration.
- ✓ Praise profusely your child if he/she adopts good manners.
- ✓ Never scold your child at the dinning table.
- ✓ Also, don't indulge yourself in arguing with your spouse or kids at the dinning table.

## Chapter Twenty Nine

### Protect your Skin in winter

During the winter months, skin normally becomes very dry and parched and even cracked. Everybody needs to care about their lips, fingers, knuckles and the corners of their mouth.

How you can maintain the moisture levels of your skin in winter season

Most people enjoyably love to stroll in chilly winter. It is the season not only of wearing the warm clothes and having fireside reading and moreover snuggling close to the pillows wrapped from head to toe with comfy quilt but it is a pleasant season to share warm feelings of comfort and joy with friends, kids and family also.

But for some ladies who are casual to the care of their skins, winter means something much more sinister for them.

Needless to say, dry skins, runny noses, cracked lips and rough hands will tell you the sorry story of how much insincere you are towards the protection of your skin.

If you are not alert for your skin protection, not only your lips and cheeks take a beating during the cold months but your feet, scalp and hands also will wear rough patches.

Here, there are some favorable tips which may assure you to get rid of itchy, flaky skin in winter and keep the wintry troubles at bay.

## Use oil based moisturizer

It is much important to moisturize your skin to keep it from flaking and feeling dry all the time. For it, it is better if you choose some good quality oil based moisturizers instead of any water based moistening product.

Oil based moisturizers will prepare your skin in better way to brave the winter specific conditions. But be alert, always choose non-clogging oil based moisturizers because generally oil based moisturizers clog up pores. Such moisturizers can instead harm your body.

## Avoid the excessive use of hot water

Generally, in winter, ladies use hot water while taking shower to brave the wintry atmosphere but the excessive use of hot not only drying out the skin but it harms to both the scalp and hair also. Warm water decreases the natural oils of the skin. To make your hair moisturized and moreover silky and sleek, always use conditioner preferably.

To restore the softness of scalp and the hair, moderate massage of your hair with aloe vera or olive oil works wonders. It reinforces the moisture to your hair. Generally beauticians advise ladies to treat their hair with olive oil massage once or twice in a week from root to tip.

But, those who have already oily hair; should massage into the end of their hairs. It is better if you heat the oil before its use and moreover, allow it to soak in a time lesser than the time you take in summer season.

Don't soak your hair in oil for long time otherwise it may cause fever.

Some ladies prefer herbal oil to soak their hair in winter. No doubt, it is a wonder substance for the softness of hair and the scalp but herbal oils are more suitable for the summer as such oils have cooling ingredients.

Don't soak it for long time. They may give you fever. Never use hot water to wash your hair. It will dry your skin and hair. Even blow dryer can hang out to dry your scalp. Wash your skin with fresh and cool water. If there is chilly winter, use lukewarm water. The excessive use of hot water may look your skin older and desiccated inviting wrinkles.

## Drink sufficient water

Don't forget, the texture of your skin depends not only on external treatments but also on the nutrients and water intake. Sufficient water, juicy fruits and proper nutritious intake also help in rejuvenating your skin from within. Most of all, the water plays an important role in keeping the skin alive and supple.

It has proved that a good amount of water helps in retaining the moisture of skin as well as keeping skin's disorder at bay. Fruits and green vegetables in diets will give sufficient water to the body.

No doubt, in winter, it is difficult to drink cold water; you can take lukewarm water or hot green tea. With water, your body will get the same hydration. Moreover, antioxidants in green tea will help your body to stay healthy.

## Wear woolen clothes

Don't be careless while you go outside in winter night or in the chilly morning. Be sure to cover up your skin. Don't let the freezing temperatures and harsh winds dry your skin. Wear gloves, scarves, jacket etc. to keep the cruel weather away from your body.

Some ladies prefer to wear silk scarf. You can also wear silk fabrics if you are endurable to chilly winds at late night marriages functions. Woolen clothing like hats and scarves can damage to your hairline.

In marriage ceremonies, you can avoid it. Also, try keeping your hair away from being open and wild. Ladies! Don't let play rough on your hair. Fashion connoisseurs suggest that ladies can style their hair with a smart braid, twist or a knot which will make their looks elegant as well as they will be able to protect their hair from chilly winds.

## Common precautions

1.   Must use cold cream on your face and lip balm on your lips before going to office and at night before going to bed.
2.   Use the paste of ground green gram powder instead of soap to make your skin soft and supple or you can use creamy soap which renders your skin extra suppleness.

3       Pamper your skin with coconut oil before taking bath to heal the dryness of your skin.

4       Must apply good quality body lotion on your entire body thrice in a week or massage your body thrice in a week.

5       Add some drops of mustard oil to the water before you are taking bath. It will help retain the moisture lost when you take bath.

6       If your lips are cracked, dry or chapped, use lip balm, petroleum jelly or Vaseline to protect them. Don't lick your lips repeatedly because your saliva will chap your lips more. Butter is also an effective treatment in curing chapped lips and rendering them an extra softness.

7       When you need to immerse your hands in water for long time, wear rubber gloves to protect its skin. Don't forget to use a base coat over your nails against cold weather.

8       If your lips are constantly dry and chapped, after taking a shower, take an old toothbrush and gently rub its bristles across your lips and remove the dry skin. After completion, use lip balm onto your lips to get them moisturized.

9       In winter, due to wearing shoes and boots, generally, the heels of the ladies tend to become dry and cracked. For its protection, you need to soak your feet in a mixture of warm water, salt and baking soda for at least five ten minutes. After soaking, rub your heels with hard stones and scrub off the dead skin.

## Skin Care: Tips @Home Fruity care

1       Not only you eat fruits, use them for your skin beauty in winter. If you have some papaya or a

bunch of grapes in your fridge, take some of them, smash them into a pulp and place the pulp on your face for almost twenty minutes. Then, wash your face with lukewarm water. Within minutes, you will have a refreshed face.

2      You can try to beautify your skin by adding five teaspoons of honey with two tea spoons of carrot juice.

## Salty care

First exfoliate and then moisturize your skin with sea salt by adding olive oil. Mix ¾ cup of olive oil in 3 cups of sea salt. You can also add some drops of your favourite oil for scent. Rose and lavender oils are great choice for relaxation. While getting into shower, rub the salt brush onto your dry skin and feel as it exfoliates. Have a plenty of oil in your hand also so as the scrubbing doesn't ache you. Simply rinse off the mixture in the shower or you can bathe in the salts but don't use soap when you rinse.

## Care with brewed tea

If your feet are stinky by wearing winter boots or shoes, it is simple method to get rid of the bad smell just with wasted brewed tea. Let the generic brewed tea cooled into the bin.

Then, soak your feet in the tea for at least 15-20 minutes to remove the bad stinky smell. Then you rinse off your feet with some water and shoes too and then you will discover that you are getting rid of it forever.

## Cuticles care with honey and lukewarm water

The mixture of one cup of warm water with one teaspoon honey and two teaspoons lemon juice is best treatment for cuticles care. Soak your fingers at least 15-20 minutes in the water. It will make your skin softer and better. Then you can gently push away the dead skin from around your nail and the tips of the fingers. To polish off, massage a moisturizer around each cuticle.

## Chapter Thirty

### Care Your Lips in winter

In winter, we observe that our lips get chapped and dry. The change in climate affects the skin of the lips which is the most delicate area of our body.

The cold weather evaporates the moisture of the lips causing the lips to dry out. The main reason of the lips becoming dry is dehydration, wind exposure and licking the lips. The best way to prevent and treat chapped lips is to keep the lips well moisturized all the times

Needless to say that chapped lips are painful and sometimes, they turn glowingly red and began to bleed due to cracking and peeling of the skin. Moreover, they become too sensitive and feel rough. The most worrying factor is that it fractures your smile.

There are several reasons such as exposure to chilly wind, vitamin deficiencies, obstructed breathing, fungal infection, dermatitis and use of harsh skin care products that lead to the lips getting chapped, dry and parched.

In winter, we generally tend to lick the lips to make them wet and soft but after some time; they again become dry and chapped as the wetness evaporates.

The saliva strips away the natural protective oils of the lips leaving them dry and sore. Smoking is also one of the reasons that lead to rough, chapped and dried lips as smoking strips the lips of its natural protective oils.

## How to prevent dryness exfoliation

Doctors, in general, advise that one should exfoliate the lips to prevent its dryness. Although, they are not parched, yet you must exfoliate its skin at least once a week to remove the dead skin cells which make the lips rough and dry.

A simple way to exfoliate the lip is to use an old toothbrush with mild exfoliating product, run your lips gently with the toothbrush, using the exfoliating product for a few minutes.

## Apply lip balm or Vaseline

The markets are flooded with several lip balms but try and use a product which contains the maximum moisturizing ingredients and natural oils.

Good quality lips balms contain nourishing ingredients and emollients which soothe and nourish rough and chapped lips. They also offer sun protection and protect the delicate skin of your lips from harmful UBA and UVB rays.

Apart from lips balms, petroleum jelly, Vaseline, lip glosses and creamy lipsticks are also available in the markets for the care of your lips. If you are using Vaseline, rub it on your lips gently once or twice a day, not repeatedly.

All these products work greatly for soothing dry, chapped lips as they lock the moisture in the lips.

## Points: Never to Forget

- ✓ The best way to chapped lips is to stop licking your lips.
- ✓ Lip balm can be used whenever you want. It can't damage your lips. Use vaseline only twice a day.
- ✓ To remove the dryness, quit smoking.
- ✓ Never use any lip product which contains salicylic acid.
- ✓ Never exfoliate your lips if they are bleeding or if there is an infection on your lips.
- ✓ Drink plenty of water to keep your body and skin hydrated.
- ✓ Keep the air in your home humid. It will remain your body and skin moistened.
- ✓ Whenever you go out, apply lip gloss, creamy lipstick or lip balm on your lips. It will help your lips to fight against the wind.
- ✓ If the wind is chilly, cover your lips with scarf and protect it.
- ✓ Cracks at the corners of the lip may be the reason of vitamin B deficiency. Consult the doctor for deficiencies' supplements.

## Chapter Thirty One

### Care Your Hair in Monsoon

Dripping hair during rainy season gives the ladies a sexy look. It is the time for enjoying the rain dance. But do you know hair suffers the maximum during rainy season. Constant drenching in the rain may cause a number of scalp problems apart from the hair loss

If you have oily hair, then the problem is colossal. High humidity can affect your hair enormously loosing its shine, making the hair dull, limp and lifeless due to chlorine in the rainwater.

Moreover, during monsoon, perspiration on the scalp also invites dirt and pollutants which are harmful for both the skin and the hair.

It is the salt in the sweat which, mixing with environmental dust makes the hair rough and bad. So, during rainy season, you need to take more care of your hair and skin.

### Don't Forget

1   Wash your hair with shampoo which suits your hair type.
2   But before its use, don't forget to rinse your hair thrice to remove the fungal growth and lice breed.
3   If hair is oily or frizzy, it is better you use shampoo frequently until the monsoon season ends. Henna conditioner is ideal for all hair types.

4    Apply the white of an egg before shampoo at least half an hour to quickly reduce the oiliness.

5    Tea and lemon are also good conditioning agents which help in reducing the oiliness.

6    Never use too many styling products which can invite dirt and pollutants.

7    Try to protect your hair from constant rain water protecting yourself from lice infestation. Rainy season is the breeding time for lice. Remember, hygiene conscious person also can become the victim of lice infection in rainy season.

8    Before stepping out, dry your hair fully. You can use the hair dryer but it is advisable you keep the device at least eight inches away from the hair.

9    Moisture can cause dandruff. During rainy season, hairs are prone to dandruff which later becomes the reason of hair loss.

10    To protect your hair from "Pus filled boils" on your scalp which causes severely painful and irritating itching, it is better you use shampoo which contains Betadine AD.

11    If you are planning to colour, perm or style your hair, don't do until the monsoon ends. Such treatments don't yield good results during rainy season.

12    If you are prone to fungal infections, consult your dermatologist for medicated shampoo. Some people say that washing hair with shampoo may cause hair loss. It is an outdated idea; discard it as early as possible.

13    If your hair is exposed to rain everyday, wash your hair everyday also with mild shampoo. If you already have some skin problem then must consider the reactions before applying chemical shampoo onto your hair.

14      Don't tie up your hair when they are wet. They will break because wet hair tends to break very easily.

15      Comb your hair with wide toothed comb.

16      If it is necessary for you to style your hair during monsoon season, use humidity protective gel for protection. Non sticky hair spray also can be used for extra protection.

17      Last but not least keep your hair and scalp nourished with high protein diets containing olive oil, eggs, whole grains and nuts. Biotin stimulates the hair growth rapidly. Drink plenty of water also.

## Chapter Thirty Two

## Scent of Seduction

Do you know the fragrance of your body attracts the opposite sex? A good fragrance always enhances the mood. So, don't let your body be smelt badly. Always honour your body by applying scent of good quality of any brand

It is a hundred percent true that both men and women are passionately attracted towards fragrance to enhance their mood. Women with a nice fragrance catch the attention of men more than the women who do not smell good.

Since the time immemorial, fragrances have been used to induce a romantic mood and pleasant feelings. If we look back at Egyptian history, those people knew the secrets and power of smell and fragrance. Fragrance was then used for mood enhancement and romantic enticement.

This secret was passed down through the ages and even today, fragrance is used to arouse the sense of smell and delight. Obviously, all women and men wish their opposite sex to notice them so when they go for any get-to-gather, they use fragrance to increase their appeal.

That is why; the perfume industry has always been thriving. Undeniably, in recent times, every woman from any stratum of society; loves to use perfume because it makes her feel seductive. Moreover, it gives her the feelings of being a complete woman and makes her confident.

## History beckons

Perfume, a Latin phrase; is the combination of two words. "Per" means thorough and "fumes" means smoke. Initially, the pleasant smell which drifted through the air from burning incense was known as perfume so; the first meaning of the perfume is incense.

Incense was first discovered by Mesopotamians about four thousand years ago. Egyptians carried perfume with them from birth until their death and sometimes, they put perfume in their tombs to keep them fragrant after death.

At that time, perfume shops were popular places where people liked to congregate. This is said that the Greeks were trained experts in the art of making perfumes which were quite different from the ones available in the market today.

That time, perfumes were fragrant powders mixed with heavy oils, devoid of alcohol. History says that Cleopatra- the famous and beautiful ruler of Egypt too was well acquainted with the power of scent and was generous in the use of perfume.

By the beginning of 20th century, most perfumes were prepared with natural animal or plant ingredients. To have such a perfume was a luxury at the time. With the introduction of synthetic ingredients, it became more accessible to everyone.

The first synthetic fragrance was created from coal tar. Fashion connoisseurs say that in earlier times, perfumes and colognes were not widely used by the common people as they don't know their benefits. Initially, the technique of preparing fragrances was discovered in ancient Egypt. Later, Romans and Arabs improved upon it.

## Benefits of using perfumes

Perfumes have been used for centuries. It is a luxury and not a necessity. In both ancient and modern times, it has proved itself to be a valuable commodity. Despite being a luxury, its popularity is growing. The reason is obvious: the wearer of perfumes gains delight and happiness by using it.

Each scent whether it is natural or synthetic emits molecules which penetrate the nasal passages and eventually reach the olfactory epithelium. This part of the nose has receptor neurons covering with nasal hairs known as cilia. Cilia catch the fragrance and gives message to the brain and to decide as to which one is good for the entire body.

Several researches say that the ingredients used in perfumes such as ginger, Jasmine, mimosa, patchouli, wood, fruits, vegetables, herbs, sandalwood and rose improve our concentration by triggering stimulating effects on brain neurons.

This increased stimulation which is augmented by the use of perfume assists in our everyday assignments. It improves our stamina and energy for focused study. It is also helpful in improving our immune system.

Certain scents have calming effects on our brain and some scents help reduce anxiety and tension. Lavender and Bergamot are such kinds of perfumes which have been used for centuries for this purpose.

Above all, perfumes make the wearer feel fresh, relaxed, cool, pleasant, gorgeous and attractive. It makes you feel good about yourself the all day.

If you are attending a party without wearing a quality perfume, you will feel yourself as an incomplete woman. By wearing a perfume, we feel confident and it is definitely beneficial.

## Negative effects of its overuse

Without doubt, perfumes do a lot good for the wearer but they are not always good for all skin types. It actually consists of a variety of synthetic chemicals that are manufactured in laboratories. Many perfume ingredients are far from natural.
If they are worn for occasionally, they are good but their overuse can affect the skin harmfully. There are several types of perfumes which are available in the markets but branded are good quality ones. They are safer to use. So, always buy good quality perfumes.

Remember, your skin and beauty is more precious than money. Generally, the chemicals, which are used in perfumes, have adverse effects on skins. Take some precautions before buying perfumes for you.

1      Check if the perfume is good for your skin. Some people have very sensitive and are more prone to rashes and allergies. Don't buy the perfume results in an allergic reaction.

2      Overuse of any perfume even if it is famous can cause instant headaches, dizziness, nausea and mood swings.

3      Scented chemicals aggravate lung diseases. Their overuse and repetitive application can worsen lung disease.

4       Its' repetitive and overuse can lead to asthmatics attacks also.

5       It is a scientific proven truth that there is a close connection between memory and scent. Due to excessive use of perfumes, the chemical fragrances can cross the blood brain barrier and cause neurotoxicity affecting the brain tissues.

6       By wearing excessive perfume, their fragrant chemicals may penetrate the skin and enter into the blood stream. They may travel inside the body in the blood stream and affect any part of the body that is sensitive to chemicals.

7       The excessive use of perfumes can also affect the eyes and concentration.

8       Never wear the perfume which the others are using.

9       If you have complaints of asthma or any type of allergies, don't use any kind of perfume

**Which scent you need to wear?**

Perfumes smell different on different people. There is no guarantee that; what smells good on someone will smell the same if you wear it. It is your own perception and taste which may help you to decide the right perfume for you. Never wear a scent which you don't like a bit. Let your intuition give you a signal as to which perfume matches the chemistry of your skin. So, never choose a same type of scent repeatedly. Replace it from time to time according to your mood, season and occasions. In hot weather, perfumes with natural scents are quite better. When you are going to office, ensure that you use a light fragrance with a light floral note. Remember some points.

1    If you are extrovert, active, optimistic person, wear flower and citrus scents.

2    If you are an introvert, oriental scents may be right for you.

3    If you are emotionally charged i.e. sensitive, dreamy and romantic, aldehyde flower scents will suit your perfectly.

## Some Tips to Remember

Perfumes may be fun to wear if you remember some tips while buying and wearing perfumes.

- ✓ Don't buy any perfume without trying a sample. Wear it at least ten minutes before deciding if you like it. This will allow the alcohol to evaporate and the oil of perfume will interact with your skin oils; then you will be able to choose your perfume.
- ✓ Always try a sample in the late afternoons because at that time the power of smell is stronger than that of morning time.
- ✓ Don't rub the wrists together while you are trying a sample. It reduces the effects of the perfumes.
- ✓ When you are trying a sample, wear perfume on pulse points such as on inner wrists; jaw line near the ears or backside of the knees are better places to send out the scents.
- ✓ When you are thinking of a new perfume, always use it on one small area of the skin.  If there is an allergy to any of its chemicals, it is the safest way to find it. Wait for at least an hour; if there is no reaction, the perfume is safe to wear.

- ✓ Don't apply perfume to clothes or jewelry. It may cause stains on them.
- ✓ Always store the perfume in a dark, cool place to keep fresh longer. Interaction of sun light and heat with perfumes' oil can reduce its effectiveness.
- ✓ Don't wear the same perfume throughout the year. Changing temperatures affect its scent.
- ✓ In cold temperatures, wear stronger scents because cold reduces its intensity within short period.
- ✓ In summer season, wear lighter scents to get rid of the bees. They can be lured to perfume mistaking it for flowers.
- ✓ Don't use the same perfume for more than two years.

## Chapter Thirty Three

### Stylish With Tattoos Carefully

These days, the trend of exhibiting tattoos on different parts of the body, both by men and women, is in vogue. Today, more than ever before people are getting tattoos done. It has become a passion for all beauty conscious- single or married, young or old.

Needless to say tattoos are regarded as a symbol of love, beauty, peace and romance etc. There is a multiple range of tattoo designs- sacred hearts, angel wings, butterflies, birds, scorpion, names of lovers ones etc. but girls particularly love to get those tattoos which make them look feminine, beautiful and sexy

Some girls might like complicated designs; while others choose common and simple tattoos depending upon their individual emotional choice and fashion sense.

Ladies generally get tattoos on their arms, shoulders, legs; both upper and lower backs etc. If you meet girls, they would say it is a great way to attract others' attention. In big cities, it has become a trend to use these pictograms to express love and emotions for someone special.

### What is tattoo and how it is marked

Tattoo is a design which is imprinted with the help of small disposable needles and different types of inks. With the help of needles, tattoo experts inject the ink into the dermis or the lower layer of the skin.

It is an art which has now become globally popular. The

word- "tattoo" has come from "tatua" which means "to mark". For centuries, this form of art has been used by the people of all cultures and countries.

In the olden times, decorating the skin with beautiful tattoos was a popular practice, but that time, the method was quite different. At that time the tattoos were marked with needles or pointed knives by hand; but now electric machines are used to mark tattoos.

In India, not only it has gained social acceptance but it has become a style statement for all generations also. In fact, I personally don't favour tattoos but if you want to be done it, be cautious and contact the experts.

If you are planning to remove the tattoos after a short period, it is better you avoid it because its removal is very painful and risky because the dermis (the lower layer of the skin) doesn't flake away unlike the epidermis (the upper layer of skin)

**Stylish tattoos to attract attention**

If we look back the history of tattoos, even a few years back, tattoos were rarely seen. At that time, it was considered as an exception and a rebellious fashion statement of young generation.

But in the last twenty years or so, the scenario has rapidly changed. In fact today, tattoos are widely accepted and have become popular both among ladies and men. Indian cinema and TV serials promoted this fashion widely.

We still remember when Saif Ali Khan had Kareena Kapoor's name tattooed on his arm and became the lover boy in the eyes of Indian young generation. So, it is the best way to attract the attention of others.

Certainly, stylish women and girls get tattoos marked on their skin to attract people's attention. So, the trend of large size tattoos that have eye catching designs or shapes is now-a-days the latest craze.

Girls often say that they love to get large tattoos marked on their back so as to show off to their friends when they go swimming.

Moreover, when I work out at the college gym, girls notice the beauty on my back. When they ask me about, I feel delighted. Once a college girl (who had asked me not to disclose her name) told me that she has a tattoo marked on her right arm. It looks beautiful when she wears sleeveless shirts, boys look at her and friends discuss her tattoos. It is a delightful experience and she enjoys it very much.

 So, if you want to be stylish like that girl, go ahead and have the tattoos made the way you want. They will definitely serve you as memories of lifetime but

I again advise you to be very careful in finding experts. In the market, there are different kinds of tattoos available. As for costs, the range is from Rs: 200 to Rs: 15000-20000. Here are some important types of tattoos:

**Japanese Tattoos**

Traditional Japanese tattoos have a special demand among girls. These are designs with Japanese characters; each character denotes a particular meaning.

Apart from this, girls love to have dragon, carp and fish

etc. which are large enough to cover their backs or arms.

The most significant feature of Japanese tattoos is that they create a delicate balance of power and beauty providing designs that fit into anybody's personal style whether they are different and complex.

**Tattoos for men**

Although, more women love to have tattoos than men, yet men make different fashion statements by getting tattoos on their chests, arms, forearms, neck and calves etc. They don't tend to hide the love they have for someone special.

Such tattoo loving people are amazed when they see a tattoo emerge onto their body parts. They go mad with joy when they get a sketch don.

In face, they are able to make more sense of their emotions through a tattoo than any other vague symbol. Girls are different as they want an excuse to show off their body.

Girls like to get tattoos on their lower backs, ankles, shoulders, upper backs, and rarely on their stomach or chest as they have to consider the parts they cannot show off with their tattoos during a formal event.

**Be cautious**

Tattoos is a modern fashion loved by all generations but before you get tattoos on any part of your body, you must be cautious, otherwise, you may lose the beauty of that part of your body and skin.

✓ Whether you go to a salon or a beauty parlour, keep in mind that you must keep the tattoo designs dry and clean away from sunlight.

✓ You must decide how long the tattoo will stay on your body. If you feel any pain or the tattoo causes an allergy, contact a dermatologist.

✓ Always be careful while choosing the tattoo and the entire procedure.

✓ Clean your tattoos regularly and use any dye free mild product. You can use fragrance free body lotion for keeping the skin around the tattoos soft.

✓ Don't soak the part in hot water for at least the first two weeks and avoid swimming.

✓ Don't let the soap stay on your tattoo. Remove it with water as quickly as you can.

✓ The ultra violet rays of the sun are the enemy of tattoos. So, avoid exposing your tattoos to the sunlight but if it is essential to go out in the sun, use sunscreen effectively.

✓ During the process of healing, tattoos start itching, if it is so, neither pick it nor scratch the tattoos, just slap the area and apply lotion to get rid of itching.

✓ Don't get a tattoo over a mole. It can produce a cancerous mole growth.

✓ Always visit a reputed tattoo artiste. Tattoos made by inexperienced persons can cause skin problems such as red bumps due to inflammation or allergic reactions. Such allergic reactions can occur even years after tattoo was made.

✓ Always follow the doctor's advice. Carelessness may put you in the danger of getting diseases like AIDS, Hepatitis B, tetanus etc.

## Each tattoo bears a symbolic meaning:

✓ Heart tattoo represents the emotions of romance and love

✓ Flower tattoo signifies natural beauty and feminine exclusivities.

✓ Butterfly stands for simplicity, peace, new life and new beginning.

✓ Star tattoos represent the glow and excellence of gorgeousness.

## Chapter Thirty Four

## Make Your Skin Sleek and Beautiful

Healthy body, wealthy busts and glowing skin with rosy cheeks is what every girl and woman desires to own. Women generally fantasy to look like gorgeous film actresses or soap opera's stars. They are often worried, when they find traces of red, angry pimples on their cheeks. They run from one clinic to another and try to seek every remedy to get rid of their arch foes.

No doubt, pimples vanish with time, but eventually, the skin loses its charms and sparkle, Dermatologists say that women's skin is more sensitive than that of men's. It ages rapidly than men's. And the skin on the face is even more susceptible than that of the rest of the body.

However, one should not forget that oily skin is much better than other skin types, though it is prone to acnes, pimples and other skin diseases. It ages at a comparatively slower rate and is also slower in showing wrinkles and yellowing. Here are a few tips to take care of the oily skin, protecting it from pimples and other diseases.

### Tips to follow

- ✓ Don't wash your face several times a day. Too much of washing forces the skin to release more oil, resulting in the gradual desiccation of the moderate skin.
- ✓ Don't use harsh products. They cause the loss of the body's natural oil. To compensate it, the oil glands

have to work overtime. Moreover, it caused flakiness in the body.
- ✓ Don't use skincare products which make your skin feel taut. They can shrink the upper layer of the skin, deterring the flow of oil into skin pores.
- ✓ Always try to keep the pores unclogged. For cleansing the skin, always use lukewarm water with good quality soap.
- ✓ Don't ever use alcohol based cleansers or lotions.
- ✓ Always try an anti-bacterial lotion or medicated soap for cleansing.

## Skin treatment in winter

Skin needs constant moisture. In winter, generally, the oil glands begin to produce less lubrication. There is sufficient loss in oil as well as sweat glands. This loss of moisture makes the skin dry, coarse and rough.

Sometimes, it cracks the skin. Dry skin is common in lower legs, thighs, elbows, feet etc. It mars the beauty of the body. Here are some simple methods to get back the glow of your skin.

- ✓ Apply a blend of one teaspoonful warm olive oil with some drops of glycerin and some drops of lime juice, at least once a day.
- ✓ Mash half a ripe banana, add some honey to it and make it into a paste. Apply it on your face; then wash the face with cold water. It will rejuvenate the glow and radiance of your face.
- ✓ Take some fresh cow milk, not boiled. Rub down mildly with cotton onto your face. Let it dry for 15-20 minutes. Then wash with fresh water.

✓ Prepare a mixture with cucumber juice, lime juice and rose water. Wash your face with the mixture. Apply the mixture on face all night. In the morning, rinse your face with fresh water.
✓ Simply applying milk twice a day can also keep the dry skin at bay. Keep it on for at least 10 minutes; then wash your face with cold water.
✓ Mix one teaspoonful milk cream with 2-3 drops of lime juice. Apply this mixture and leave it for minimum 10 minutes, before taking bath.
✓ Khus- Khus (poppy seeds) is a magic elixir in protecting the dryness of skin. Soak 100 gm khus-khus overnight. Grind it in the morning, adding some milk, to make a paste. Apply the paste on your face; wash with fresh cold water. It will revitalize your skin miraculously.

## Organic treatment

According to Dermatologists, the botanical ingredients in skincare treatment are magical. It is a natural concept of skin cure. Medical experiments show that our body responds positively to organic treatments.

The application of fruit acids to the skin has showed spectacular results. Its consistent use results in considerable decline in the rough distortions of the skin surface.

No only does it make our appearance fine, but also removes the wrinkles amazingly. Organic treatments don't have any side effects. They are absolutely non-toxic.

Vitamins work like magic in skincare. Vitamin A revives the radiance of the skin. It gives the skin suppleness and agility. Vitamin B stimulates moisture absorption.

Vitamin C controls wrinkling and gives freshness to the body. Vitamin E is a fantastic medicine in minimizing the scars and wrinkles; so, the creams and lotions having Vitamin E inputs are sold maximum in the market. Despite that, do remember, just buying several medicines or tons of make-up lotions and creams to hide the damage is not a permanent solution.

## Method for having silky, supple and lustrous skin

1. Always eat a balanced diet. Proper diet is more effective than the lotions or creams. What you put into your body will reflect on your skin.
2. Always take proper sleep. Lack of sleep will make your skin look older. 6-8 hours sleep is moderate. Night going parties' butterflies always leave dark circles under the eyes. I suggest such ladies to have a sound sleep.
3. A regular yoga or exercise routine must be scheduled to remain fit and healthy.
4. Drink water as much as you can. One jug or two or more. Water gives the skin suppleness and protects your skin from being dehydrated.
5. Exfoliate two three times a week to clear your skin from dead cells.
6. Inhale fresh air deeply, to give a new look to your skin. Exposure to cold wind can also harm your skin. Differentiate well between fresh air and cold wind.

7. Don't expose your skin in the sun. The damage done by the ultra-violet rays is highly risky and can not be reversed easily.
8. Normally, use plain water for washing your skin, if there is no dust on it. Maximum use of soap or cleaners damages the skin. It gives dryness to the skin.

**Beauty glimpses from kitchen: Groundnut oil:**

Blend one teaspoonful groundnut oil with five to six drops of lime juice. Apply the mixture on your face and see wonders- how pimples and blackheads run off from your face.

**Almond:**  Almond is a boon for dry skin. Grin two to three almonds daily, mix them in honey. Apply it on your face regularly and notice the charm and freshness on your face. Almond oil can also be used for dry skin. Almond is also helpful in removing old pimples.

**Apples:** Apple juice is best for cracked skin, inflammations and itches. When it is applied on the face, you can see your wrinkles slowly and slowly begin to remove.

**Drumsticks:** Drumstick helps in eradicating black spots, blackheads and pimples. A mixture of grounded drumstick past with limejuice is the best medicine for skin ailments.

**Cucumber**: Apply the juice of cucumber with carrot or lettuce juice to cure skin breakouts. You can rub cucumber on your face also.

**Garlic**: Rub raw garlic on your face for persistent pimples. You can use it with puffed rice also, to reduce skin infections.

**Fenugreek:** Applying the paste of fresh fenugreek leaves on your face, before night sleep, and washing it off with warm water in the morning is a moderate medicine to prevent pimples, blackheads, wrinkles etc.

## Chapter Thirty Five

### Choose the Right Sneakers!

Characteristically, sneakers are of three types- straight, semi-curved and curved. One can determine the type of your foot shape by looking at the bottom of the shoes and verify the degree of pronation.

If you have flat feet or low arch, straight types are the right choice for you. If you have medium-height arch, semi curved shoes are satisfactory for you but if you have high arch, you can ideally opt for a curved shoe.

Without determining the shape of the foot, one can invite blisters, calluses and injuries. Even straight shape of the shoe can also affect the toe very much if it is unfit to wear.

Most good shoe companies prepare the sizes of shoes on the basis of wet test or sand test experiments, so as to make the grip of the shoe strong. Cheaper shoes seem to be quite fit initially but actually, after a day or two, their grip begins to weaken and customers feel uncomfortable while wearing such shoes. Their feet begin to slip afar.

### Two pairs of sneakers

Shoe connoisseurs advise that one should buy at least two pairs of shoes. If not possible, they should replace them after six or less months. Sneakers are generally used for exercises and brisk walking, which can cause a lot of wear and tear in the shoes loosening its strong grip.

So, one should buy at least two pairs of sneakers and use them the alternate day. In summer season, one must wash the sneakers after a week to avoid the itching on the feet.

## Follow the expert's suggestions

- One should buy the sneakers in the late afternoon or evening when the feet are swollen at their largest end after the day's workout.
- If you are used to wearing socks with the shoes, wear it while buying the sneakers.
- Bring old shoes with you when you are shopping for new ones. Your old sneakers will give the ideas of degree of pronation of your feet to the shopkeepers and they will be able to check the number of your wearing shoes.
- Avoid buying the latest fad shoes. They may be experimental fashion shoes. Maybe, they remain unfit while you run or walk briskly.
- Generally, both the feet are different. Left foot is often slightly larger than the right one. Buy the actual size which is quite fit in the larger foot.
- Ensure that there is enough space for the toe by pressing the thump into the shoe just above the longest toe. Your thumb should fit between the end of the toe and the top of the sneakers and there must be half inch of space between them.

## Important points

- Your shoe should neither be tight nor should it slide around. It must be fit snugly without slipping up or down while you walk or tread briskly.

- Your sneakers should never press any area of your foot tightly. It should be comfortable from all sides.
- Some shoe shops have a treadmill; others let the customers bounce up and down. Check your sneakers with some walking or jumping before buying them.
- Your socks apart from the sneakers must also be smooth and well fitted to prevent blistering.
- Buy the sneakers from a quality shop or specialty store if you are unaware of the model/number of type you need. Specialty stores can provide you the correct type of sneakers based on your foot type and your stride pattern.
- Essentially, if you are participating in athletics and wish to buy sneaker for that especially, never wear new sneakers when you are just going for the race.

## Measure your shoe size in standing-up position

Before buying the shoes you must feel that the shoes you are buying are in action, only then you are the successful buyer. So, it is very important to measure the shoe size in standing up position and not by relaxing on the chair.

Our feet are flattened out a bit when they are under the weight of the body. They become slightly bigger on standing up. Walk some steps after wearing the shoes to check its hold. For moments, also slightly bend your knees to ascertain the comfort of the shoes.

Remember, the purpose of your buying the sneakers. You are buying shoes for just strolling or for only office duty; if they are for office duty, your choice should be different.

Always remember your running shoe size should be more up to a size than what you think your office shoe size should be.

## Precaution regarding laces

Sneakers are generally laces shoes; so be alert while exercising. Tying the laces tightly can cause damage to the nerves on the top of your feet. In good quality sneakers, stiffer foam on the upper part or in the tongue of the sneakers is used. Only buy good quality shoes, which will be helpful in protecting your nerves in the foot.

## Seek help from shopkeeper

If you are not sure regarding the model or type which fits you best, seek the help of shopkeepers. Often shopkeepers are not just salespersons, but are experts. They might ask you several questions like, how long you run/walk briskly everyday, how much do you weigh or regarding your foot problem, if any. Tell him everything correctly; he will definitely help you in finding a right model of shoes/sneakers for you.

## Different sneakers for different type feet

Experts suggest particular types/model of shoes for different type of feet. For flat feet or over pronate, they suggest motion control running sneakers, as these are supportive in controlling to prevent the feet from rolling in too far and its straight shape give your feet the maximum support.

They are also known as control-oriented running sneakers also. For high arched feet or under pronate, you can opt for cushioned running sneakers.

These types let the feet roll inward. Its curved shape encourages the foot in motion. Its soft mid sole helps us in comforting the bottom of the feet.

Stability running shoes are helpful for those who have normal aches. Such types of sneakers offer a good blend of cushioning and durability. Generally, such sneakers are of semi curved shapes. They don't control the foot motion as rigorously as motion control sneakers.

## Care for your sneakers

Good quality sneakers are expensive. If we remain slapdash regarding their care they will lose its strength. Follow the tips how to care about your expensive sneakers.

- If your sneakers become dirty, wash them with hands using sponge or cotton swab. Machine wash is harmful for them. Commercial shoe products also can be used for washing them.
- If your sneakers have become wet, put wrapped newspapers inside them to quicken up the drying.
- If you have bought the sneakers only for running or walking briskly, use them only for these purposes. They will last long and won't smell due to regular use.

# Section II

# Happy Life

## Chapter Thirty Six

### How to Make Women Good Friends

The attraction for opposite sex is natural whether you are at your workplace or in any recreational club; most men feel neglected when the ladies they are trying to befriend don't respond favorably.

Obviously, such men don't have the qualities their female colleagues and friends want to see in them; consequently, they are unsuccessful to command the respect of ladies.

The significant question is: what exactly is that the ladies actually want in men. What are the exceptional qualities they wish to see in their male colleagues, partners or friends?

Normally, we see men behaving slightly different in the presence of their female colleagues just to make an impression on them but phony behaviour actually doesn't work for long.

Here are some tips for men to know how they can impress their female friends or colleagues and make them their true friends for life.

### Build confidence

Undoubtedly, most working women like men with good looks, decent manners and broadmindedness. These qualities attract the women, but if you lack self confidence (which is considered as the best quality) you may be unable to impress your female friends.

Thus, to begin with, have confidence in yourself. If you are nervous while expressing your viewpoint to your lady friend or female colleague, you will not impress her. Instead, you may become the laughing stock for your female friends. Apart from good looks and decent manners, generally, ladies are attracted to those men who look confident. Snobbishly rich and overconfident men upset ladies.

So, always be comfortable in any situation to delight your lady friends and colleagues. Remember, being confident is strikingly an attractive point. It may make you more attractive than you really are!

## Get groomed

Grooming is also one of the best ways to impress others. So, you must pay some attention towards your grooming also. It's not about visiting a beauty salon every week or fortnight. It's all about a regular morning shower and shaving before going to your place of work.

After the shaving is over; you must apply cologne on your cheeks to soothe them. Dress elegantly and stylishly. Don't put on the same dress for two three days continuously.

Generally, ladies take notice of such things. Polish your shoes daily; dirt on them won't give a good impression about your personality. If you wear necktie, its knot should never be slacking.

In general, ladies prefer those guys who take care of themselves and look great. Most women do not like such men who have a bushy back, unkempt beard, fat gut, dirty teeth and sullen face look.

Usually, they are turned off by body odour also. So, for the sake your lady friend, if you really wish to stay with her; buy a good quality deodorant and use it regularly. In a nutshell, you should look like a gentleman. Women like to befriend with handsome and groomed guys.

**Listen to her adoringly**

When some lady in whom you are interested in, begins to talk to you, show some curiosity about the things she is talking about. Listen to her with full attention as if, for you, nothing is important than her and your life depends upon the story she is narrating.

Let her tell you about her dreams, experiences, feeling etc. Let all your assignments or engagements be neglected for some time. Ask encouraging questions, showing interest in her conversations, which will attract her towards you.

Whenever, she asks questions; respond with a smile and see in her eyes deeply. An excellent idea would be to express flattering remarks, which might also draw her attention towards you.

When you are talking to her, ask her opinion about your decisions. If she says something, then, value her viewpoints with a pleasant smile.

After that, you need not wait for her; instead she will begin to call you and greet you frequently. Always remember that ladies detest those men who don't listen to them attentively. It annoys them; so listen to them attentively.

## No sleazy attitude

Ladies love attention. If you listen to her attentively, they feel delighted. While talking to women, most men habitually move their eyes on their body parts.

Some pervert guys think that a woman's body starts from neck down and they focus there which is embarrassing for both of them. Ladies have extreme disgust for such males. They enjoy talking with those guys who pay attention to their mind and emotions instead of their body parts.

If you say a word of admiration about her beautiful eyes or a mole over her lips; she will take it as a compliment and smile in response but if you say a word of praise for her breasts or some other similar body part, she will get angry. So, while talking to your lady friend, don't utter a sleazy remark ever and never speak about her private body parts.

Moreover, constant praise is always a bonus point. Don't praise her only once or twice. You must pay her a compliment every now and then, offer her a drink; invite her to your chamber during lunch break.

But, be careful, don't let the people know you are interesting in her otherwise she will take no interest in you. No woman wants to be the centre of attention of people around her.

## Always respect her

Women are generally more emotional compared to men. They feel wounded if someone misbehaves with them publicly. Sometimes, there might be a difference of opinion between you and your lady friend or she might deserve to be reprimanded for some particular reason but don't reproach her publicly.

This might spoil your relationship. If you are rude, ignorant and don't know how to behave with her in public, get yourself trained in etiquette some way. If you tend to repeat such behaviour regularly, you would be split from her and in most cases, she will avoid you like a curse. So, understand her, respect her and always be humble to make her a good friend forever.

## No boredom please

Women love listening to funny stories. They respond readily to conversation. They like men who have funny stories to tell and who can make them laugh.

So, don't tell her your sad, long monologue or stories of your dismal past. Avoid sharing with her your broken relationships with other friends. Women generally don't like listening to boring, uninterested stories. They always want to be happy and like cheerful friends. If you are a singer, sing to delight her.

If you know how to play a guitar, you must use it while singing. Singing is always a soothing balm for ladies.

## Looking handsome and neatly clean

Ladies, in general, detest speaking to those men who look dirty or grubby. They have a special nose to catch the disgusting odour coming from men's bodies. So, always be neat and clean. While visiting women, don't forget to groom yourself completely.

First, make your hair good-looking and utterly touchable by using anti-dandruff shampoo. Second, keep your finger and toe nail well trimmed and clean.

Always keep your nail short and cut straight. Don't smoke before visiting lady friends. If it is a habit and you cannot kick it off, clean your lips and put mouthwash candy or peppermint to freshen up your breath.

Some men are naturally hairy. They have hair on their back, chest, ear, neck and on their eyebrows. If you have hair coming out of ears, nose or through your T-Shirt, it looks very messy. Trim those unwanted hair as early as possible. Ladies don't like the "grizzly bears" as their friends. Have a tweezer with you to pluck the hair if it suddenly comes out of your nose.

## Don't' be freak

At workplace, some men madly run after lady colleagues to impress them. They invite them over tea or request to watch movies with them. Cordial relationship with lady colleagues in offices are welcome but if a lady doesn't respond to your tea invitation favourably, don't force her to accompany you.

Such freak practice can give a bad impact to your career and family. Women like etiquettes and self-respect. If you force her repeatedly, even your words of praise for her will not have value for her.

## Treat delicately

In office, if your lady friend asks you for a special treat on a special occasion of your birthday or marriage anniversary or your promotion, don't ever show that you are short of money. Accept the challenge.

Give her special party. She may ask you to take her to a nearby restaurant with some other lady colleagues, don't hesitate to spend on them. Remember, if you spend money on a woman, she feels that you really appreciate her.

Also, be careful towards the bill. Don't scrutinise it when it reaches you and also don't question the waiter or restaurant authority regarding the high cost of cuisine. Just a quick glance on the bill is sufficient.

Remember, ladies don't like such friends who are stingy with money and haggle with the waiters over the bill.

## What the ladies want from men

- ✓ Men should ask about her interests, work, hobbies and family.
- ✓ Men should listen to her attentively and give respect to their opinions.
- ✓ Men should always be honest, truthful, friendly and sincere towards them.

- ✓ Men should keep their promises intact. Don't make false promises.
- ✓ Men should always refrain from vague boasting.

## Chapter Thirty Seven

### Aqua Exercise: A Cool Fad to Keep Fit

Are you a fitness freak, bored with traditional gym exercises and looking for different physical-training to keep yourself fit? If your answer is "yes", then here is some good news for you: a new variety of gym, Acqa Gym, is gaining popularity, and some say it is better than the traditional gym for various reasons

Gone are the days when fitness freaks used to adhere to ground gym only. More and more people are now taking to water exercises or water therapy, not only to stay fit, but also to get rid of body ailments.

Once an employee at the Aqua Spa Club, Bangkok told me that, now more and more wealthy men and sophisticated women from all around the world are turning to aqua therapy, as these exercises, definitely, not only tone muscles, but also give life to the heart and lungs, and help you beat the stress and anxiety.

Water is cooler than body temperature. Hence, people have to labour hard to keep themselves warm in water. It's really a good point about aqua activities. Moreover, it's not necessary for you to know swimming. Even without knowing it, you can do what you want and get cured of your ailments.

In aqua exercises, the only equipment required is water. Trainers say that water demands twelve times more resistance than air, while exercising in a pool; so, they claim that one water exercise is equal to ten ground ones. If you run on ground you will burn eight calories in a minute but in water exercises, you will burn up 12 or more calories in a minute.

## Floating equipments

Moreover, if you want to do multiple exercises simultaneously, you cannot do them on floor; but, you can do that in water with the help of floating equipments. With floating equipments, you can even perform aerobics without the fear of knuckle injuries or drowning.

Aqua Gyms are always recommended in high water, so that the exercise freaks may open up their body parts freely, with their full vigour.

## What is aquatic therapy?

It is a kind of water healing to soothe your body. Some say, it's a water exercise also. Any exercise or any type of activity which is performed inside the water is referred to as "Aquatic Therapy", either it is for enjoyment and fun, or for health.

So, experts split water activities in two parts, relating to both exercise and sport, and fitness and health. First, it means that any exercise performed in water is to continue your regular exercise routine. Second, any type of "beneath-the-water" exercise is to recover from a serious injury or any other ailment.

## Expert's opinion

Tim Tift, chairman of Physical Education Department at University of California once said that, "since I started aqua jogging, I have decreased my body fat from 24 percent to 14 percent, in a little more than one year. With the practice, his metabolism was up, and he felt a lot better, as if he was revitalized. In America, people preferred water therapy, as compared to India, because of the lack of facilities in aqua gyms. Data says that more than 2.2 million people have discovered the benefits of running in deep water in America. More people are expected to take it up in the future.

A basic aspect of exercises in water is that you can exercise without undergoing the jarring sensations that you generally experience when you exercise in a ground gym.

At the time of running or jogging, when the heels or knuckles accidentally touch the ground, the weight of the body is intensified up to five times, and you find your ligaments badly bruised; but during aquatic exercises, you don't ever face such a situation.

Water will always allow you to perform exercises without any hindrance. That is why, doctors always recommend pregnant women and senior citizens to join aquatic activities rather than ground exercises, as they are risk-free, cool and enjoyable. Water is cooler; so the body temperature is always restored. There is no chance of fatigue or perspiration in water.

Even in water, aerobic activities are performed without any risk for the knuckles. Sometimes, injuries, orthopedic conditions, back-pain and excess weight don't allow people to perform exercises at gym.

For them, exercise in water is a great solution, for fitness and recovery. In aquatic exercises, water gives a beneficial massage, which is useful for blood circulation and melting of adipose cells.

## Breaking the monotony

Exercise at gym is a traditional idea. By water exercises, you can not only break the monotony, but also involve all your body muscles in the exercises, as they all work against the resistance.

Moreover, such exercises will benefit you on cardiovascular, muscular and flexibility level. Everybody can perform while exercising in water. Water will make your body lighter, neutralizing gravity.

It would give huge support to your ankles and knees, and other parts of the body. What is more, it's a unique idea to break the boredom of ground gym exercises.

### *Aqua jogging*

Jogging in water is more enjoyable than jogging on the ground. It is a non-weight bearing activity and doesn't affect on bones, ligaments, tendons etc. Since your feet don't touch the bottom in deep water, you are able to get all the benefits of the toughest aerobics activity in water.

Not only jogging, but all types of exercises in deep water are among the fastest growing trends in India.

Health-oriented people of every age are taking advantage of this stress-busting fun, not only for burning their fat but for toning their muscle, recovering from their injuries and restoring their sluggish cardiovascular systems also, all for a small payment.

But, aquatic therapy is not about paddling up and down your vicinity pool, or relaxing in a bubbling hot spa; it is much more than that.

## A boon for sporty person

If you are an athlete or sportsperson, and you are accidentally injured due to ground exercise, and if you still want to participate in the upcoming events, in such cases too, aqua exercises are very useful. Through aqua gym, sportspersons can do their regular practice.

Moreover, others who work out regularly have chances of minor injuries during an exercise session, but in water exercises, there are fewest chances of being bruised; rather, they assist in recovery.

## Advantages of aqua exercise

Aquatic therapy also helps you in the following ways.

1      It's helpful in heart diseases and hypertension.
2      It increases muscular strength
3      It is the safest exercise for pregnant women.

4       It improves the alignment of posture, balance and co-ordination
5       It is the safest exercise for overweight people.
6       It increases the flexibility of muscles
7       It improves the range of mobility in the body
8       The muscles experience a soothing, massaging effect.
9       If the weather is very hot, you can practice in a lake/pool outdoors. If the weather is very cold, you can opt for a heated indoor pool. In both situations, you are able to do your exercises.
10      The coolness of water attracts all; and so, everybody enjoys such experiences.

## Chapter Thirty Eight

### Making Each Moment Pleasant

Do you know the worth of spousal relationship? Healthy relationship with the spouse makes the life quite enjoyable, worthy, pleasant and lovely. No doubt, you must have your prime duty towards your family, kids and work, but in these responsibilities and hectic job schedules, never forget your own needs and mellow moments.

Make a balance between your duties and relationship. Worship your relationship and make the each moment of your life malleable and pleasant to delight your mood and make your life happy

In India, there are numerous families which are more focused on children than on themselves. There are two types of couples, one children centric couples, two spouse centric couples. Sharing out between two is a better option, if you love to be healthy, vivacious and fresh. Bedrooms are the likes of spas, if you indulge in activities freely and unworriedly.

It is natural that when children are born, loads of responsibilities come up. Couples discard sex, then, as an unwanted aspect of their lives. They rarely have considerable time for each other, in sharing rich moments in their bedrooms.

In such a drastically changed situation, sometimes, they look like roommates more than husband wife. Such a situation is really detrimental, both for the couples and their families. Such couples are prone to a series of diseases. Medical study suggests that, for healthy mind and physical beauty bedroom exercises have significant importance.

However, here are a few tips which will, for sure, revive your relationships and zip up your bond, if it is near to split. Believe it! Acting upon them will truly benefit the miserable couples in saving their relationship as well as the sacrosanct institution of marriage.

## Don't forget to plan a day

Planning in everything is essential. So, plan your day for sex too and don't drop it even if you are terribly busy. Some may laugh listening to this odd idea of fixing the day for sex, as we all know that it's entirely a spontaneous activity. But, actually, it also can be pre-planned.

Discard this myth propagated by movies and fictional novels that sex is just spontaneous, not planned. It, for sure, can be planned if you choose a day for yourself and determine to work for it to happen.

Make up your mind essentially. As the scheduled day closes by, you will feel an enormous sensation inside your body. Even psychiatrists advise sex for at least twice a week, which is the need of the body, if you wish to be fresh, healthy and good natured.

Undeniably, it's a kind of "keeping-fit exercise" and is a genuine one to meet the body's needs. Fixing a day doesn't make you sound like a maniac couple; rather, it is a praiseworthy one.

These days, couples' lives are so intensely busy that, if you don't fix a schedule to connect sexually, you probably won't find a time for it, and it won't happen by itself.

## Don't let anybody know your plan

Lovemaking is a secret issue and it should always be. So, don't let your friends or colleagues about your plan or the scheduled sex day. If you let them know innocently or frankly, probably, they will mock at you and spread rumours in the office, which can humiliate you immensely.

Sex with full energy, interest and enthusiasm is an investment as your relationship gets energized. Marriage is a solemn commitment to your partner, and regular, unhampered, delightful and luxuriant sex is a shield for protection of your marriage.

It's a totally personal thing in your life. Sharing your spouse's sexual activities with friends will be as shameful as sharing your spouse's body with them. So, don't embarrass yourselves.

## No movie, no dining out

On the fixed day, abandon all other activities or programmes, which can hinder your enjoyment. Instead, concentrate on decorating your bedroom with different kinds of flowers, petals and perfumes. Refresh your room with room fresher scents. Replace your bed sheets and pillow covers. Prepare yourself as you are going to win over the heart of a prince/princess.

Cool your bedroom with AC. Don't go out for a movie or dinner with friends or relatives on that particular day, come what may, as you may get tired and late. Sex should not be taken as a procedural task.

Enjoy it with your full enthusiasm and interest. Prolong it as long as possible. A light music in your bedroom during romps can heighten the pleasure. Every organ of your body will sing a song of pleasure, if your partner's soft hands touch it amorously.

Send your kids over to their grandparents' or friends' home. Talk lovingly with your partner all day. Don't wrangle over domestic help or kids' study.

Stay at home the whole day; if not possible, return from office as early as you can. Postpone all your other assignments and preserve all your energy and time for the main course. Dine with comfort. Sip your drinks enjoyably.

## Avoid begging

There are two types of partners. One who possesses a higher drive for sex, two- who avoids sex either this way or that way, i.e. they have lower drive for sexual activities.

The former one, more often than not; desire for lovemaking, in different ways and at different times. Be it the soft moment of night or the clamour of the day activities, they thirst for sexual pleasure, all the time.

If the schedule is fixed, they might not be able to ask their partner for frequent sex, as they would themselves feel plagued by the risk of rejection. Begging or pleading dies down the very purpose of sex and the emotions of intimacy behind it.

When a couple agrees on a scheduled sex, it's presumed that it would happen at that very time, the very day; there should be no reason for stopping it.

But that doesn't mean that you are not allowed for occasional spontaneous romp. If you are in the midst of hills, and cool breeze touches your silky body, may be your partner ask you for lovemaking behind the shrubs, don't let go waste of such wild, memorable moments of intimacy in the relationship.

**Cool down the brain**

The most sensitive organ of the body is the mind, which manages the all physical activities. If you set up your date for sex, it (brain) would begin to work specially for it. It would boost your desire and augment your happiness as the moment closes by.

Of course, the partner who has higher sex drive wouldn't have any hitch in making the bedroom a playground of sexual games any time.

But those- who are deficient in sex drive, too might prepare themselves for the date, because they would be required to adhere to the commitment. Fixation of date would act as a catalyst to the process, and the couple would prepare themselves mentally for being together.

Brain gives us the mood to play and also readies the low-sex-drive. It would always make your enjoyment unforgettable. Always cool down your brain to meet the date.

## Goal towards intimacy

Fixing a date for sex does what the couple most needs, creates intimacy between them. Some couples complain that they reach home after ten, and then dine, so, how they can create storm in bed despite the day being the sex date. Their hectic schedules and workload doesn't allow them pounding a sexual tornado in bed with their partners.

Sex on the calendar helps the spouses in reminding that they should work together to achieve the goal of their mutual intimacy. 'Fixed sex date' values couple's emotions for each other. It's a promise that should be fulfilled.

## Stick to calendar

Sex is an unpreventable marital recreation. Preplanned sex reminds the spouses of their goal of enjoying life and being healthy, apart from other assignments and the burden of family, kids and workplace responsibilities. The calendar sex programme makes the couple the lifetime learning of awarding pleasure to each other.

It also gives the partner a sense of togetherness. If the couple is annoyed with each other, the upcoming date would gradually, cool down their anger. No doubt, sex date gives the couple an opportunity to 'must sex' but it doesn't mean that, on the other days, it should be prohibited. Sex is spontaneous as well as scheduled.

## Accommodating the need

Sex whether it's at daytime or at night, gives pleasure, if it is done with freedom and co-operation from both sides. It's a reciprocal activity. One partner may prefer lovemaking at night, while the other may fancy during the day, behind the faint darkness of fabric sheets. If you wish to do the activity two times a week, you can choose one session at daytime and the other at nighttime.

Couples, in general, differ with each other, both over the frequency of sex and its atmosphere, which is congenial to them. Some have no schedule, and whenever they seek opportunity or find no kids around in the vicinity, they indulge in the activity. Fixation of date for lovemaking would accommodate the need of both the partners and they might not wrangle over such a delicate issue. They definitely would not behave like hungry monsters.

## Prepare yourself fully

Every day is important, if it's in your calendar. Sex is the most subtle issue; if you fail enjoying it fully, it will hurt your heart. So, be fully prepared to do lovemaking with your partner. Scheduling sex will prepare your mind to be ready for the enjoyable activity.

Don't miss it. Take a shower at evening, scrub good smelling lotion onto your cheeks; beautify your body at parlour. Do all that can spice up your enjoyment? If you are fatigued much and lacking in lovemaking, first take some; then go to your bed.

Honoring your commitment with your partner will deepen the trust and intimacy in your relationship. If some problem arises on the fixed date, then, you can fix another date, or opt for an alternate plan to meet your physical and emotional needs. The key motto is: enjoy sex and be healthy.

## Chapter Thirty Nine

## Gym at Home

Because of loads of assignments and busy work schedule, we generally have to sit before computer long hours regularly. Our diet during working hours also becomes irregular and most of us depend only on junk, unhealthy and imbalanced diet.

The result we all know; we have to undergo the miserable experiences of flabbiness, stress and obesity. To avoid such a situation and keep yourself fit and healthy, gym at your home is the need of the hour

To keep themselves healthy and fit, most of us plan of visiting the gym but due to busy schedules and hectic lifestyle, they find themselves unable to step out of their homes for that particular purpose.

Believe it or not, recently, most of us have adopted an unhealthy lifestyle without much thought only due to irregular exercise. Actually, we have become so lazy that even walking, cycling etc seems to be an enormous burden on us. In such a scenario, none can protect us from the evils of several ailments if we remain failed to exercise regularly.

Have you ever thought about home gym? It's an alternative medium of exercising at home, at your convenience. Establishing a tiny gym at home is an ideal option to get into shape, without stepping out of home.

If you have your personal gym, you need not abandon the comfort of home and reorganize your work schedule. Follow your prearranged schedule, and sweat out whenever time allows you in doing so. To save on time and to maintain regularity, having a home gym is the most happening trend of the contemporary times.

## Professional help is must

Before establishing a gym at home, you must contact an expert or professional coach for you. Also, talk the family doctor or instructor to know about your physical needs and endurance level for different sort of exercises at your home gym. Initially, seek guidance from well trained professionals; otherwise, you will probably do more harm to your body than benefiting it. And you may also not get the desired results.

If you have sufficient disposable income, then it is not a bad idea to hire a personal professional coach or trainer for you at home, for some time.

Most professional coaches charge about 8000-10000 per month, and visit the home gym as per clients' requirements. They give their clients a personalized diet chart and its schedule. Generally, coaches give 60-90 minutes to their clients per day, as per their requirements.

Home gym must not be huge and space consuming, but as simple as it can be. A combination of warm-up and cardio-vascular exercise machines, along with weight training equipments are moderately enough in a gym at home.

## Respect your health

The first and most important equipment we need for our personal gym is a treadmill. Warms up, jogging, running and walking briskly are initial steps before we start an exercise to shed the excess body fat. With the treadmill, one can do these activities at various inclines. With the help of a cross trainer or a rowing machine equipment, one can also do different sorts of exercises for the movements of their arms as well as legs. This is ideal equipment for a complete workout and for toning muscles.

Sanjeev Marshal, my trainer friend opines that today most people love to buy only treadmills. This is only equipment which can be used for several purposes. Treadmills are available in the market in different models.

If you prefer a non-motorized treadmill, you have to pay less, but have to labour hard while motorized treadmills are expensive, but have more features. I must suggest you to buy good quality equipments to keep your health fit and well. The more you respect your health, the more you enjoy your life.

## For entire family

Remember that, physical fitness is not a fad. It's our necessity in these times when our life style has absolutely changed. If you have treadmill at your home, every member of the family can enjoy the benefits of it. The women and children who are reluctant to go out for walks or jogging in unpleasant winter season, or feel shy to work out in the in the presence of strangers, gym-at-home, with only two-three equipments is ideal to meet their needs.

One can feed his/her data viz. cholesterol level, height-weight and blood pressure into the machine and see the difference after some days' work-out. Moreover, if you have a gym at home, you can save both your travel time and gym fee as well. You can burn around about 200-700 calories on treadmill.

These days, in big cities; people prefer to have their personal gym in their houses, because they know that it is only the home gym which can provide them a total body workout, including cardio, strength and flexibility.

Often people think that gyms are for youngsters; but I stress gyms are for all, young or old, children or women. Needless to say that treadmills, whether they are manual or automatic are wonderful for exercising.

Good treadmills are imported for Taiwan. When you plan to buy a quality treadmill, ask for Taiwan model.

## The concept of multi-gym

If you have no budget constraint, you can choose three equipments plus extra equipment namely the multi-gym, collectively, to make your home gym multi-purpose.

Treadmill is most important, remember it. Cross trainer, stationary bicycle and a compact unit of equipment- multi-gym extra can make your home-gym a multi-propose centre for diverse exercises, weight-lifting and jogging. It all depends on your needs.

And moreover, you must seek professional help in deciding what equipment suits your fitness needs. If a stationary bicycle is sufficient or should you buy both treadmill and cross trainer.

If the experts recommend that one machine would suffice to meet your exercising needs, then what is the purpose of buying other equipments and waste your money?

Apart from three important equipments, if you wish to tone-up your muscle, then you must buy weight-lifting also but after taking the expert's advice.

## Know your gym equipments

### Treadmill

As I have told earlier that treadmill is one of the most important equipments. On a treadmill, beneath the feet, there is a belt system. The top of the belt moves to the rear allowing the runners to run fast or walk briskly in the opposite direction.

Treadmill has become a very popular way to lose weight and burn off flab. One can burn about the same number of calories as walking or running outside. Benefits of treadmill exercise can be felt during summer when it becomes very difficult to walk outdoors.

With a treadmill in your home, you can burn about 200-700 calories. Treadmill helps in toning body muscles and maintaining overall fitness. Moreover, pregnant ladies can also do exercise with the treadmill, because it gives no side effects.

## Elliptical trainer

The word elliptical means an oval-like shape. It is an innovative technology in the world of exercise and fitness, which gives us fun along with exercise. An elliptical trainer is a stationary exercise machine which is used to replicate walking or running without putting unnecessary pressure to the joints.

The machine has footpads that allow you to stand up while exercising. To maintain balance, you can hold on handgrips. Such activity decreases the risk of impact injuries. With the help of this machine, you can do non-impact cardio-vascular workout as per the volume of the intensity of the machine.

While standing on this machine, there is little impact on your joints, unlike in treadmills or joggers. Finally, we can say that elliptical machine provides a low-impact total body workout. Generally, people do weight bearing exercise to improve bone density.

Constant elliptical motion does create a low-impact workout, which is like brisk walking. Its handles allow users to work upper body muscles, providing total body exercise.

## Stationary bicycle

The other name of a stationary bicycle is an exercise bicycle. It is a device with saddle, pedals and handlebars in the shape of a bicycle. But, it is just for the use of exercises and not for transportation. It is a good machine for cardio workouts. It has less impact on knees, hips and other joints than running or brisk walking. It can be used at any convenient time.

These are of two types: motorized and non-motorized. Motorized stationary bicycle allows the exercisers to adjust resistance and speed. It does computerized control of the speed. Meter on its front measure the volume of work done by exercisers. It is a good machine for lower body workout.

Most exercise-loving people have only stationary bicycle at home for several purposes viz. to improve cardio functions and weight-losing etc plus it's also a fun. With stationary bicycle at home, one can exercise in his convenience discarding the worries of bad weather, stray dogs or snarling traffic etc.

**While exercising at your home gym, remember these important points.**

1. First learn; then use the proper technique while using equipments.
2. Don't lift the excess weight initially itself; it can harm your body.
3. Adequate rest is essential after performing some exercise activities.
4. Breathe systematically to increase your capacity of doing some extra work.
5. Maintain proper balance, or, you may jeopardize your body parts.
6. Don't do any excess in exercise.
7. Must warm up your body before doing hard exercises, including weight-lifting and running on treadmill.
8. Never be in hurry to change/increase weights.

9.  Concentrate on a single area of your body at one time.
10. While exercising, if you experience any kind of pain, stop exercising. It can prove harmful.
11. Wear proper clothes and shoes to feel comfortable while exercising.
12. Cool down after finishing your exercise schedule; despite having several plans ahead.

## Chapter Forty

### Ageing Blues, No worries

The more you grow emotionally, physically, mentally and psychology, the more maturity comes upon you. So, value your full-blown period of growing age and make the best use of it. You can utilize your maturity in guiding your youngsters and support them in every possible way, in stead of wailing about your wrinkles or sagging flesh.

Don't forget, the autumn of life is always better than spring. If you think positively, your coming years will be full of joy and expectation. With getting old, you can be more proficient, productive and wiser.

It is time to develop more self-confidence and sharpen your skills. It does not mean that you forget your wrinkles or sagging flesh. Do take care of them, but without being bawling and weepy.

### Enjoy the independence

Almost, "after forty" is the period of enjoying independence. When the women attain this age, they must have cultivated the qualities of compassion and understanding. These qualities definitely will help them to take on the challenges ahead.

Ask yourself, are you not more complete and worthy, when your children have grown and become independent? They need not ask for your service; instead, they can be helpful to you in every sphere, even in your kitchen.

Why don't you enjoy your independence? Strands of grey hairs or wrinkles on your face symbolize your wisdom and experience of life. Take it positively.

## Cherish your dream

During their young days, women are bound to follow the rules of their elders- father in the case of unmarried girls and husbands, if they are married ones.

Dominating males are "compulsorily-stumbling-blocks" in their freedom. In such situations, their dreams generally go astray and they are forbidden from doing things to be tied down with other responsibilities that they are not able to do what they think they are competent to do.

But as they get older, they are liberated to work independently and can cherish their dreams, or devote full time to their hobbies. Longevity with the husband makes the gentleman to respect her emotions. Now, the women begin to understand what is truly important and right for them or what is wrong.

At this phase of life, even the one time "stumbling block" husband can also be helpful in realizing their partner's dream. Ladies "after forty" really can recognize their worth and hidden talent inside them.

It is the age of bringing forth their gifted talents. With the growing age, they can share their responsibilities with their grown-up children also.

## Boon phase

"After forty" is a boon phase in many ways. At this period of age, kids grow older and become more or less independent. And women can find their spare time for their hobbies. They can devote themselves to numerous types of creative activities.

If the children have gone to far flung cities for higher studies, it does not mean that they are left alone. They can share their moments of happiness or bouts of pain with the husband. Talking with kids on the mobile phone or a live chat with them on the PC is an enchanting experience.

Count yourself blessed, as you will find more spare time for the work of your interest. You can even choose a course for yourself then. So, have the courage to be different and chase your long-cherished dreams.

At this age, definitely, you will be less afraid of your failure, as you already might have gathered enough courage to brave the odds of life. Enjoy every moment of this phase. You have nothing to lose, be it pursuing a hobby or taking up tuition classes. So, dare to be different and follow your lost dreams.

## Accept the truth

Actually, each woman desires to look younger than her years. The current trend of spa treatment, massage or surgeries for attaining a youthful and beautiful look should not be accepted, despite that spa is one of the best modern techniques to uplift your mood and keeping you fit and healthy but the fact is that these techniques can not hide the age.

Age itself speaks and these techniques of beauty enhancement never erase the signs of growing old. If one tries to mask the signs of growing age, grey comes more visible. So, think for yourself; is this what you are looking for? Accept the truth and reality whatsoever.

This concept of honesty must be applied to maintain the body and soul intact, in order to live peacefully. Essentially, the focus should be above the looks and body figures. Maturity guides us to seek a deeper level of relationships and seek ways to make the life more fun and frolic, enriching and wonderful than just opt for a "face lift" or "wrinkle erasing" exercise.

## Hilarious laugh

Smiling or cracking jokes with hilarious laugh is the best known method of killing the worries, anxiety and depression. Frowning or showing your vexation can not change the world from what it is.

So, always try to discover the ways to smile, be happy and be in high spirits. Scientifically, a good laugh releases endorphins from the body, which is considered like oxygen for the body. Laughter must be an integral part of your life. Whether you are busy or free with no responsibility, make laughter your morning time hobby.

Ask yourself, is it a difficult task? Yoga or physical exercises or activities also releases endorphins hormones. If you find time to participate in physical activities then you will find double benefits. You need not join a gym for such exercises; fix your schedule at your home.

It will give you scores of benefits. Brisk walking or easy yoga exercises are enough to keep the endorphin flowing, which is essential for the wellbeing of your health and life.

## Tuning with nature

Nature is always friendly with human beings. So, one of the best and effective ways to combat the fits of depression is 'nature-healing'. Some name it "nature therapy". Tune yourself with nature.

Early morning walk in a flowery garden is one of the best ways of tryst with the nature. Adopt such an attitude and see the difference and feel the change, as to how nature sits on your lap and helps you in metamorphosing of your soul and mind.

How much is a glance at the starlit sky, when you are laying on a wooden charpoy under a dark roof, inspiring and pleasant? Have you ever tried to fathom its beauty and charm? Nature itself gives a lesson.

When the trees move their head at the command of windy air, it shows its happiness and enthusiasm. If you are pessimistic, you will relate their shaking with the ups and downs of the life. Positivism and optimism extend the delight of our life.

At sunset, a walk with your partner or friend or kid by the sea, will give you a sense of peace, contentment and serenity. The overriding waves too give us a sense of understanding. Sea does not worry if its waves come uncontrollably. Learn it and let the unpleasant things pass unperturbedly. The buzz word is: please…please no aging blues, no worries, enjoy life.

## Chapter Forty One

### Give Your Leisure Time a Great Meaning!

*If your millionaire husband doesn't want you to join any nine-to-five job despite being you are highly qualified and talented and you desire to do the job to kill your boredom, don't make yourself down in the dumps, there are several ways to keep yourself busy at home and make the life meaningful*

After kissing the husband a goodbye and sending the kids to schools, generally ladies prefer to glue on TV sets in spite of finding absolutely nothing interesting to watch. They watch the uninteresting movies or monotonous soap operas boringly to pass their time.

The question is: it is the right way to spend your leisure time at home? Why don't you make your leisure time creative and meaningful? There are several hours daily when nothing in particular is keeping you busy and you can make your leisure time meaningful by developing your hobbies? Don't forget constant sitting or your sedentary habits at home may also cause obesity and blood pressure to you. Here are a few ideas for you to kick start the fun time.

### Make your blog

One cool way of spending your leisure time is to create your blog on internet. If you have an email account at Google you can create your blog easily through blogger.com. It is one of the best popular sites for blog buffs. Apart from it, there are several sites also which provide the facilities of blogging. Even some people earn enough by allowing Google to post the advertisements on their blogs.

It is a best way to share your unique ideas, memorable photographs or video clips with friends. Through blogs, you can also meet the people of your interests and hobbies. It is a worldwide style for the display of one's ideas or calibre.

Most of the world's prominent and distinguished people-writers, journalists, models, film stars, artists, painters, photographers and even business men have created their own blogs and they enjoy sharing their ideas and creativity. Why don't you delight your mood by creating your own blogs?

## Cherish your hobby

Everyone has a hobby or passion and that may be painting, gardening, writing, pottery or music etc but most of us in the hurry of our daily engagements, forget it. Now, after the husband go off to job, you have some free time on hand to utilize it.

Why don't you cherish your hobby in leisure time and gladden yourself? Pick your creativity where you had left it and do something which you really like doing it. It would be really delightful, enjoyable and lovely to add something personal to your creativity. If you are interested in painting, you can please your hubby by creating some unique portraits for home décor. It will add so much more to your house. You can also paint a wonderful landscape for one of your best friends' drawing room. It will boost your relationship with friends.

## Exercise or yoga

At present time, our life has much strained due to several pressures and reasons. Moreover, our food habits and lifestyles have become complicated. In such a situation, exercise or yoga or both is must.

It is very important for all of us to give our body a regular exercise to keep the body fit, healthy and beautiful. If you have a gym near your house, don't delay to join in and give the free time to your health.

If you are unable to go to gym or your husband doesn't allow going to gym, you can make a tiny gym at your home with just treadmill and stationary cycle or you can start power yoga or kickboxing or simply go for a jog at home to keep yourself fit, beautiful and healthy.

Don't be plump and overweight and become the source of amusement for several. You can do exercise or yoga at your home anytime. Sure enough, you will see a dramatic change in your body and physique. Even your skin will also be glowed much.

## Take dance lesson

Being an accomplished dancer is a delightful experience. If you are interested to develop yourself into a dancer, it is a great time for you when you are alone at home without husband and kids. By being a dancer, you can impress your husband with your skill. Whenever you go to any wedding party or get-to-gather celebration and know the dance; don't forget to show off your charisma of talent. Taking dance lesson is one of the best choices for all. There are numerous dances styles such as salsa, jazz, fox trot or jive.

It entirely depends on you which style you like the most and pick it. Take dance lessons at least one month to be an expert. The best thing about dancing is: not only it rejuvenates you but gives you a total fun also. You always feel alive, young and fit. Sure enough, by taking dance lessons, you are learning a new talent and also at the same time providing your body a total workout.

## Learn a new language

Learning any new thing in itself is a great enjoyment but learning any new language is both enjoyment and a feeling of possession. When it comes to learning, it is never too late. It's a wonderful avenue. There are several ways to learn a new language. You can engage a tutor at home to teach the language. If you are interested to learn something by yourself, markets are flooded with several types of books and CDs. By buying them, you can learn the language at your home.

For it, what you require, just your willingness to learn and some time. Very soon, you will become the master of language. If you wish you enjoy the learning more, you can invite any of your friends at home and learn the language together. Apart from it, there are also so many other wonderful things that you can do at your leisure time such a swimming, cookery or art classes. Creative workshops are also there for your fun and enjoyment.

## Enjoy reading and write articles

Reading is a fun. It is a fantastic habit as well an exercise for mind. Reading makes the mind sharpened. The more you read, the more you improve your language. And, with the improved language, you can write articles on different subjects and contribute to newspapers and magazines. All in all, reading is the habit of a winner. At any time, each of us has the long list of books that we must read.

So, now; you have some extra time in hand why you don't make that list a little shorter? Make a cup of coffee or tea and curl up with latest bestseller and you will find that it is the time very well spent. For writing articles, you can get opinions from different people through your online expert friends of different areas. Moreover, you can read several types of articles to develop your own opinion.

## Meet friends for lunch

Another cool option is to get totally dolled up and step out with some friends for lunch at your favourite haunt. Each of us has a place that we love to go and our husbands and kids just can not stand that place. So, now that they are not around and you for a change have some time in hand, why not you make the best of the opportunity? Meet your friends there and indulge in some good food and a lot of girl talk. There can be nothing more entertaining and relaxing than a combination of good food and great gossip.

## Chapter Forty Two

## Smile Your Face!

*Do you know the value of smiling face? Increasing stress, anxiety and unbendable pressure have preoccupied our minds hauntingly and these days, we have completely forgotten to smile even a little. In our offices or working places, we meet our colleagues and friends casually wearing worries on our faces. Such unworthy attitude weakens our ties with colleagues and hampers the pace of our work in office*

Do you know the value of smiling face? Increasing stress, anxiety and unbendable pressure have preoccupied our minds hauntingly and these days, we have completely forgotten to smile even a little. In our offices or working places, we meet our colleagues and friends casually wearing worries on our faces. Such unworthy attitude weakens our ties with colleagues and hampers the pace of our work in office.

It is quite true, these days, down to ambitions; we are deadly busy in our homes as well as at our workplaces but it doesn't mean that we should forget to express our happiness through smiling faces while we come across friends and colleagues.

Remember, smiling is such a finest facial expression that denotes pleasure and happiness. The more we meet others with smiling face, the more we command respect and love from others. Smile, sure enough, is the beginning of the love and the pleasant emotions and moreover, it frees us from strain and worries.

## Communicate your emotions through smile

I'm of the opinion through smiles; one can communicate his/her emotions. Smile, in fact, shows that how much happy we are. Money is not everything. One can earn enough money by hard working but smile is more difficult to earn than money if it is lost. So, never let it be lost, come what may. Smiling is a simplest, easiest and cheapest ever way to build a connection among people as well as improve our looks and even moods.

It is a like a bridge between two hearts. When we frown, forty three muscles of our face have to work but if we are smiling, only seventeen muscles work to spread smiles so what is the purpose of wasting our energy by frowning. When someone smiles, his/her brain releases endorphines which makes him/her feel happy, healthy and in better condition.

## Positive attitude brings smile

If your attitude is quite positive, there is no reason, you will not be happy and in high spirits. One can't define happiness easily just in a few words. It is essentially a state of mind where we are completely satisfied with ourselves. In offices, we generally ignore our colleagues and friends due to competitive jealously. We don't meet them happily and don't smile to know about their achievements.

Remember, if you smile for sometimes, you must forget your worries and anxieties. Imagine, how a smiling child looks beautiful and sweet? Everybody loves to play with a cute smiling face child.

It is true that in a competitive life of today, it is much difficult to be happy in life but if you are happy and ever smiling face, you are blessed one. Simple point is: if your attitude is positive, you will be happy and your face always will be smiling. The art of happiness can only be achieved with positive attitude. If you are pessimistic and have a negative attitude, neither you can smile nor win in the face of harsh conditions.

## Contentment multiplies smile

Think; you are contented with yourself? If not, first of all you need to be contented with yourself. Then, it might be easy for you to smile unreservedly because contentment multiplies smile and happiness. Don't forget to smile even in your bad times.

No matter, you have bank balance in millions or every means of luxury also but if you are not contented with yourself, you will not be able to smile and in money in your bank account will not be able to bring smile on your face.

## Help others and be happy

If you help others in the times of their need, you will bring smile not only on your faces but put a smile on other's faces also. With my experience in life, I can say that by helping elders and treating everyone equally creates a positive impact on others and you can make them smile with your helping hands.

Smile is contagious. It is such a great thing which can be done as a part of our normal routine and cost nothing. By helping others with smiling face, you will be surprised to see how many people are encouraged by your kindness and support.

So, don't let insatiability and self-interest rule your heart ever. Always meet everyone with a smile on your face because it is the only smile which begins love.

## How to bring smile on others' face

1   Give someone an inspirational book to read and then see how miraculously you have brought smile on his/her face.

2   When he/she reads the book, he/she will think of you.

3   Write a hand written encouraging note for someone to give him/her inspiration and show him/her or send him/her by post. You will see a permanent smile on his/her face when you see him/her the next time.

4   Deliver a meal or tea to someone at the time of their need when he/she is sick and at bed rest. When he/she comes out of the bed, he/she will always greet you with a beauteous smile.

5   Don't forget to thank anyone who helps you at your requests or at the time of your needs to view smile on his/her face in future.

6   Always reveal a genuine smile to everyone you meet. Then, you will see how easy it is to get others to smile.

## Chapter Forty Three

## Green Time for You!

*Maybe, you are enormously aware about your health. You may also visit the gym regularly, sweat out on treadmill, attend the yoga class, go on no-carb diets, prefer to crunch salad, veggie and various fruits but have you ever thought over discovering some green time for yourself and connected to nature?*

Think, how many times in a week you go to park and glance at the greenery, sweet-smelling flowers or walk barefoot on green grass.

If you are not regular park goers, discover some time for yourself to sit in the lap of serene nature or deck your home with varieties of greenery. It will give you great relaxation and joy having great health benefits as well.

Reading an interesting book or watching comedy show on TV can reduce the stress level, but walking on the green grass or nearby the river and watching the flocks of twittering birds will give you extra pleasure also.

Roaming in the greenery disconnects one from all social and human contacts and this is an extra benefit one gets from nature.

Non green activities such as reading a book or watching the TV show can not help us in disconnecting from human relations as they are also connected to human activities.

We have to listen to the dialogues of characters while watching TV Show and read about the points of logic of fictional characters of the novel. Hence, these recreational activities don't give us the health benefits which we get from greenery.

When you go in the park, you will sense the tremendous effect of greenery on life. Human being is indeed a social animal. A small fraction of disconnection from worldly or social life can do wonders for him in eradicating the stress.

Frances Ming Kuo, a researcher at the University of Illinois had once said that greenery and nature helps not only to improve physical health but it perks up the health of mind also.

No doubt, living or wandering in greener areas is good in every way. Moreover, it is much better if you create some greener areas in the vicinity of your living place. People living in greener areas are reported to have lower blood pressures, lower stress levels and faster post-surgery recovery.

I talked to several Shimla based doctors and learnt from them that patients in Himachal Pradesh (which is a greener area) are generally better equipped to cope with the stress as compared to those patients who comes from Delhi or plain areas. No doubt, nature is an incredible healer. It can boost our mental energies.

Even having a fish aquarium in our office or at our home gives us therapeutic experiences. I also learnt from my doctor friends that people of greener areas have fewer mood swings than the people coming from non-green area like Delhi and Rajasthan and other plain states.

Walking on green grass is incredibly beneficial for us. Walking barefoot on grass not only gives us a cool feeling but it strengthens our toes and feet. It tones up our legs. It is also helpful for the bone structure of the leg also. Walking barefoot is an effective remedy to get rid of the problem of flat feet. Deformity of toes can be recovered completely through walking barefoot on green grass. Moreover, walking barefoot on grass is also helpful for respiratory system.

People residing in green areas are motivated by themselves to awake early for a morning walk or exercise. It helps us in getting rid of the ailments of blood pressure and stress plus herb plants have numerous benefits apart from adding flavour to our cooked dishes and salads but people living in congested areas are not motivated to go for walks and they experience unhealthy lifestyle.

Doctors generally prescribe heart patients a regular walk in park because it has proved that walking reduces the risk of cardiac arrest by 50 percent. Although, you are stress free, yet you must resort to greenery otherwise your sedentary lifestyles will give invitation to obesity and several ailments.

To take green benefits you may resort to green gym where you can play outdoor games and have a fun with friends. Believe it or not' green gym is better choice than conventional gym observing the health benefits of greenery.

## In Conclusion...

*As we come to the close of this book, the thought uppermost in your mind would obviously be as to how we should play our role as parents* **When our preteen daughter insists upon dating.**

Relationship analyst and the author of the popular book 'For Young Women Only' Shaaunti Feldhahn has once said that the boys and the girls are naturally attracted to one another. It is a common feeling between both sexes which generally starts in preteens.

Although, at this age, kids don't know what dating means yet they are interested in the opposite gender and want someone special to treat them emotionally and physically in a special way. Let's try to know, in such situations how we should cope with our preteen daughters?

Seema and Anjali were close friends before marriage. They also studied in the same school till 12th standard and enjoyed the same room at hostel. Fortunately, they both got married in the same city and their friendship continued.

There husbands and kids too became friends. Seema has now a 12- year beautiful daughter and Anjali is a proud mother of a 17- year old son. Due to their long standing friendship, they visited each other frequently and let their kids enjoy freedom for several hours.

One day, Seema noticed her daughter sitting on the lap of Anjali's on. She was shocked and began to spank the daughter in the presence of Anjali and her husband. Then the daughter threatened the mother that she would commit suicide if she was not allowed to go on dates with the boy whenever she wished.

She also outspokenly declared that she would celebrate her birthday with the boy because she loved him. It is not just this one case; these are numerous such cases of preteen girls dating their boyfriends.

Such trend is prevalent not only in the metros but in the small cities and township also thanks to new born smartly stylish media and emotion provoking soap operas which are nowadays shown on TV.

So, if you are the parents of a preteen daughter, do pay attention to her. Have you noticed any unusual activities of your daughter at home or school? Have you ever met her school teachers to know about her progress in the school? Have you ever observed with whom she goes to watch movies? If not, then you are not careful enough and in case your daughter goes astray, you alone will be responsible.

### Analyst's views

Relationship analyst and the author of the popular book 'For Young Women Only' Shaaunti Feldhahn had once said that the boys and the girls are naturally attracted to one another. It is a common feeling between both sexes which generally starts in preteens.

Although, at this age, kids don't know what dating means yet they are interested in the opposite gender and want someone special to treat them emotionally and physically in a special way.

Children of preteen age often have the tendency of mimicking what they see on the TV and in the movies but they still don't have a full grasp of how a relationship works. In such situations, parents should have an important role to play to control and guide the emotions of their preteen kids.

Generally, the parents have a tendency to dismiss these early relationships as trivial but they should take them seriously because it is an advanced signal of what is yet to come and it should be addressed by the parents with the help and guidance of the teachers as early as possible.

**Points to remember for parents**

When the parents chat with their children, they should make them aware of the values and expectations of their family and in the meantime, also lay out the boundaries of the family their background and provide them the reasons of these boundaries.

In spite of imposing rules, the parents should sympathetically and compassionately help the preteens to understand the reasons why the rules are there and why the parents are there to guide them.

## Mom's role to handle the situation

If you are a mother whose preteen daughter enjoys the company of boyfriend for dating or for loafing about for several hours, take it seriously and handle the case patiently.

- ✓ Never scream at your daughter when she announces that she is going to watch movie with her boyfriend. Let her go with a smile but teach her to take care of her in case of any problem.
- ✓ Never beat her in order to mend her ways. Beating may make her more stubborn and adamant.
- ✓ Never taunt her with ill words or speak to her rudely but listen to her with calmness and try to understand her point of view.
- ✓ Behave with your daughter sympathetically and caringly.
- ✓ Be a considerate and loving mother to control her emotions otherwise you may lose the love, trust and respect of your daughter forever.
- ✓ Never behave rudely with your daughter's close friends also.
- ✓ Don't blame the other girls whose company your daughter enjoys for the faults of your daughter.
- ✓ Don't impose your self-made solutions and decisions, but ask your daughter to suggest the solution for her emotional crisis.
- ✓ Don't provoke your husband to register police complaint against the boy. Don't accuse him for not caring the daughter properly.
- ✓ Don't call the boy's friends for enquiry and publicise the episode of your daughter's dating

- ✓ Don't call up the boy's parents immediately and shame them for the fault of your daughter or the boy.
- ✓ Never visit any astrologer or palmist to find solution. They are unable to give any solution except for misguiding and charging hefty fees.
- ✓ Don't call your daughter's classmates for enquiry and don't humiliate your daughter in front of her classmates.
- ✓ To conclude, try to understand the emotional feelings of your daughter. Explain to her about attraction and other facts related to sex education. Tell her that sexual behaviour at this age is a premature agenda. To instill social and family values into her mind, constant counseling is important. Fill her mind with good thoughts.
- ✓ Never let the antagonism come in the way of love between parents and daughter.
- ✓ Retain the trust and respect of your daughter for you and the family.

## Papa's role to handle the situation

Generally, fathers resort to silence over the daughter's problems and refuse to speak to the daughter about it. They ask their wives to handle the situation while keeping an eye on daughter activities.

If the wife raves and rants, he starts staying away from home giving work as his excuse. Even if the daughter talks about meeting her boyfriend at home or outside, then he doesn't take her feelings very seriously.

In desperation, upon seeing the situation going out of hand, he sometimes, begins to drink more usual. Being a responsible father, don't be laidback about your daughter and never exhibit your unsavoury attitude.

The duty of the father of a girl is to console his upset wife. It is perfectly natural for any mother in this situation to be a little anxious. In such a situation if the father doesn't help his wife to deal with the crisis calmly, he doesn't play the role of a father commendably. Another duty of the father is that he should have a quiet, firm conversation with daughter and the family of the boy and his siblings also. He should spend more time with the family and daughter and ask the other kids to notice the dating girl's activities.

He should buy some books on the subject of adolescent behaviour of kids and give to the daughter to read. He should handle the emotions of his daughter constructively by discussing with wife, family, friends etc.

If the need comes, it will be better if he consults with a professional. He should motivate the girl's siblings to understand the predicament of their sister and talk to her about the baffling feelings by serving as the bridge between the parents and the dating girl.

**A little advice to preteen dating girl**

- ✓ Try to understand that twelve or thirteen is not the age for dating or seeking boyfriends. At such a tender age, mind is not ready to handle intimate activities. Moreover, it is the age for studies and development. Let your body and mind grow. Don't think of a relationship with any boy until you gain maturity.

✓ Don't think your mother as your enemy. She is afraid of what may happen to you because she knows you are far too vulnerable at this time in your life.

✓ When your elder siblings pooh-pooh you, don't take it otherwise. They want you to learn from mistakes you are doing.

✓ When your father resorts to silence or withdraws, it is not because he doesn't care about you but because he is confused and does not know how to tackle the situation. Therefore, help your father to understand you. Don't hoodwink your parents. You still have a long life ahead. There are many relationships you will have. Just understand and value your parents' emotions.